PEDIATRIC HEAD INJURIES
A Handbook

PEDIATRIC HEAD INJURIES

A HANDBOOK

By

A. LOREN AMACHER, M.D., FRCS(C)
Departments of Clinical Neurological Sciences, Surgery and Pediatrics
University of Western Ontario, and
Victoria Hospital
London, Ontario, Canada

Department of Surgery, Division of Neurosurgery
University of Connecticut
Department of Neurosurgery
Hartford Hospital
Hartford, Connecticut

WARREN H. GREEN, INC.
St. Louis, Missouri, U.S.A.

Published by

WARREN H. GREEN, INC.
8356 Olive Blvd.
St. Louis, MO 63132, U.S.A.

ISBN No. 0-87527-337-8

Printed in the United States of America

Preface

This monograph is directed to the allied health professionals. My aim is to discuss the entire spectrum of brain injury in children and adolescents, including the sequelae that may alter the child's life permanently. We shall examine the pathophysiology of head injury, why things may go wrong inside the head following head trauma, and the clinical features that occur, transient ones and those of more serious import.

The clinical material comes entirely from personal experience. For the past fifteen years it has been my unfortunate lot to look after many hundreds of children with head injuries. Every time I reckon that now I've seen everything, something new pops up. It is a continual learning experience that we shall share.

In the past decade or so, new specialties in the health care professions have spring up and many new techniques have been introduced. The rehabilitative potential for seriously injured children has increased tremendously, and we medical professionals owe our allied health professional colleagues a substantial vote of thanks. This monograph is an attempt on my part to repay part of this debt.

Some of the illustrations in this book were prepared by Diane Falk, Medical and Graphic Illustration, 13960 West Ninth Street, Zion, IL 60099.

A. Loren Amacher, M.D., FRCS(C)
Hartford, Connecticut, 1985

Contents

PEDIATRIC HEAD INJURIES
A Handbook

CHAPTER 1

Demography and Epidemiology

In all developed countries, trauma is the leading cause of death from early infancy to well on in adult life (to age 50 in the United States). More Americans die as the result of motor vehicle accidents each year than were killed in the Korean War. This holocaust does not spare children. Except for the neonatal period, death from accidents leads the list of child killers. From ages 10 through 19, accidents kill more young people than all other causes combined. In 1975, for example, nearly 24,000 children and adolescents died accidentally. Of these, 13,000 were due to vehicular crashes and 5,200 to causes such as falls, sports injuries, accidental gunshot wounds, and so on.

The carnage, of course, is not confined to developed countries; in most emerging nations the same pattern is becoming evident. Only in underdeveloped area are malnutrition and infection still holding forth as the principal killers of the young.

Deaths reflect only a small part of the picture of the incidence of trauma in the population. Precise figures are impossible to obtain, but a conservative estimate is that 13.5 percent of all children (18 years and under) sustain an injury each year that is severe enough to prompt attendance in an emergency room. In girls, the toddler stage is the most vulnerable, while boys have a bimodal peak, toddler and teenage years.

As astounding as these figures are, those relating to head injury in the pediatric population are even more chilling. In 1978, 546,000 children and adolescents were treated in emergency departments across the United States because of head injury. Males lead the parade, nearly two to one. In toddlers, 40 percent of cases of trauma involve the head, and to the school years, 20 percent of accident victims have concommitant head injury. On a per capita basis, 1 in every 100 boys and 1 in every 200 girls sustain a head injury each year. Every male child in the United States has a 19 percent probability of suffering a significant head injury by the age of 19; for girls, the figure is 11 percent. Table 1 emphasizes these figures.

Now, of course, many of these head injuries are of little long-term consequence, but if as few as one percent of head injuries leave some type of permanent residual, some 5,500 children and adolescents are crippled in some fashion by head injury every year. Intensive efforts to limit and circumvent deficit and to restore function in this huge group of accident victims are now well begun in most developed countries, and the cost of such programs is enormous. Obviously, the solution to this very real public health problem lies in prevention.

As we shall see later, there may be considerable danger in regarding *any* head injury that produces unconsciousness as a trivial event. During the years of rapid learning, even a mild concussion may interfere with the child's ability to store or retrieve new information for as long as six weeks. More severe brain injury has been described aptly as the "great leveller." In the twinkling of an eye, a child full of promise and hope may be reduced to a dependent, crippled, even vegetative, individual. The heartache and lost accomplishment that such situations imply cannot be calculated in any financial terms. The human brain is the instrument that has created everything that is good and excellent (all that is evil and base, too) in the society of Man. I often wonder when I stand at the bedside of a child whose brain has been ravaged by trauma what new idea, what new art treasure, what spectacular

TABLE 1
UNITED STATES NATIONAL ESTIMATES OF RATES OF HEAD INJURY PER 100,000 CHILDREN

Age Group	*Males*	*Females*	*Total/100,000*
Under 1 year	1,436	1,268	1,352
1–2 years	2,224	1,297	1,761
3–6 years	1,538	1,058	1,298
7–12 years	814	301	558
13–18 years	607	312	460
TOTALS	1,028	597	813

physical or mental accomplishment has been lost for all time. The problem is of epidemic proportions in our society, yet little attention has been paid to it.

Children sustain head injury from many causes, but a general pattern is discernible according to age. In the perinatal period, most injuries occur during difficult labor and deliveries. Sometimes the extraction of an infant caught tightly in the birth canal is accompanied by a reduction in blood flow to the child because of compression of the umbilical cord. If this persists for a significant period of time, irreversible damage may be done to the brain with consequences to be reviewed later (Chapter 4). Badly placed obstetrical forceps may cause fracturing of the skull, leakage of cerebrospinal fluid (CSF), tearing of cranial nerves, or direct brain damage. Frantic pulling of the torso of a baby in the breech position may tear the spinal cord. Tugging on an impacted shoulder at the pelvic outlet may easily damage the nerve trunks to the upper extremities, the well-recognized brachial plexus injuries. Fortunately, improved obstetrical techniques and pre-natal care, and the more liberal use of Cesarean section have lowered significantly the incidence of birth injuries to the central nervous system.

During early infancy, most head injuries occur as the result of falls from changing tables, from parents' arms, down stairs while crawling. In motor vehicles, improperly designed or fastened car seats are indictable culprits. Babies held in mother's lap may have their heads crushed between the dash and mom's chest in head-on collisions. Finally, a significant number of infants are intentionally injured by parents, guardians, or siblings.

In the toddler stage, most head injuries happen because of falls — from chairs, tables, down stairs, and so on. The more mobile and daring (or inquisitive, perhaps) the child becomes, the higher the perch from which he or she may tumble. Unprotected stairways are favorite targets of infants in walkers and toddlers under way in an insecure fashion. "I only took my eyes off of her for a second!" is the common lament of mothers of these accident-prone little characters. Child abuse continues apace at this age.

Once the child's sense of balance becomes secure, he starts to chase things, oblivious of any danger. He runs into the street, off of balconies, into unmoveable objects, out of windows. Scrapes and bumps are part of the young child's normal attire. Wagons and tricycles and assorted plastic go-carts go out of control, overturn, collide. The wonder is that children of this age sustain so few serious injuries. In the car, the terrible twos, threes and fours often are totally unrestrained. In a collision, they may fly about like shuttlecocks and may be thrown right out to suffer a second collision with inanimate, unforgiving objects.

Sports injuries begin to appear in the pre-school and middle childhood groups. Frequently they are passive injuries; that is, the child is a spectator injured by an object thrown or swung by someone older. Every spring I see a number of "nine-iron injuries." Dad is out in the back yard loosening up his golf swing, little miss or junior pads up behind unannounced, and dad nails the little dear right on the head on the follow-through, causing a depressed skull fracture.

Later in childhood and throughout adolescence, vehicular accidents assume a more important position as the cause of head injuries. Highspeed bicycles, motor bikes and cars collide with one another with lethal combined velocities, and when cars smash into bikes, the right-of-way or the carefulness of the bike rider is a futile issue. Sports injuries become more prevalent during this period, as well. In most organized sports nowadays, head protection is reasonably good. Yet it is incomprehensible to me that any sport would be encouraged where the head is a target of blows or is used as a battering ram.

Throughout childhood and adolescence, penetrating injuries of the skull and the orbit occur with fairly steady frequency. Accidental gun-shot wounds and perforations by sharp objects such as sticks, knives, or lawndarts are seen fairly commonly in pediatric neurosurgical practice. At some time or another, anything that can be shot, thrown or run into at speed has ended up inside the head.

This epidemiological litany is now about complete. Sobering as it is, it is frustrating not to be able to assign a precise figure to the number of dead and disabled from head injuries each year. The best I can do from extrapolation of various data is 25,000. Twenty five thousand children and adolescents die or sustain some permanent residual from head injury every year, in the United States alone. Probably, this figure is conservative.

SOURCES AND READINGS

Preventing Childhood Injuries. Ross Roundtable Report (12th), Ross Laboratories, Columbus, 1982.

CHAPTER 2

Anatomy

1. SKULL GROWTH AND MATURATION

At birth, the skull, is very thin and pliable. The plates of bone that form the calvarium are joined by fibrous synchondroses or *suture lines.* These suture lines provide mobility to the skull, and are the sites for active bone production and skull growth. Figure 1 indicates the principal suture lines and bones of the newborn skull. There are, of course, similar growth lines along the skull base and at the skull–face junctions.

The skull grows in response to brain enlargement. During the first year of life, brain volume more than doubles and by the age of two, has reached about ninety percent of its final value. Past the age of eight or nine, further increase in head circumference is due almost entirely to thickening of the skull and of the scalp. The most explosive increase in brain volume occurs during the first eight months of life.

The skull is so thin at birth that it may be cut quite easily with scissors. In fact, I often use scissors when doing craniotomies on neonates. This thinness, with the suture lines, allows the skull to mold itself into the birth canal. The skull thickens gradually and the skull bones enlarge as new bone is laid down at the suture lines. It is possible to "spring" the bones of the calvarium on one another by digital pressure until three or four months of age. But after six or seven months of age, the skull is rigid enough that when things happen to or inside the skull very rapidly, it exhibits most of the characteristics of the adult skull.

Although the suture lines usually are visible on skull x-rays throughout life, for practical purposes they are fused by mid-adolescence. Up to that point, chronically increased intracranial pressure (ICP) may cause the suture lines to separate. During such

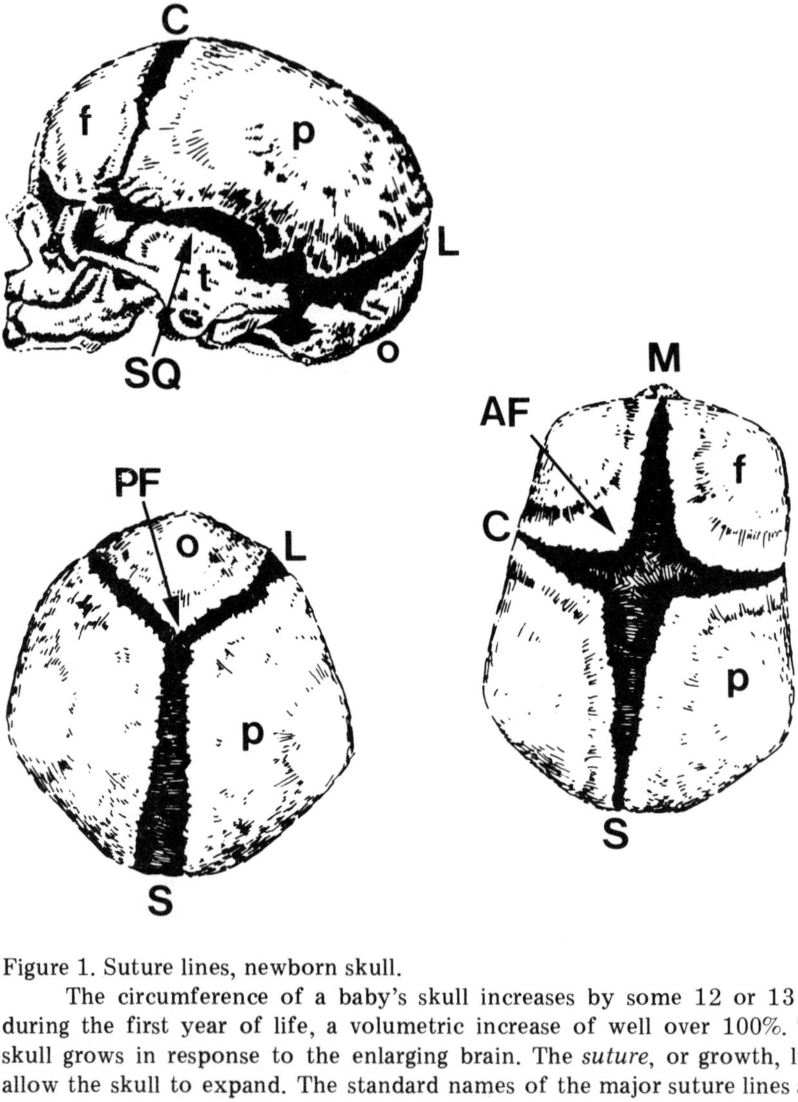

Figure 1. Suture lines, newborn skull.

The circumference of a baby's skull increases by some 12 or 13 cm during the first year of life, a volumetric increase of well over 100%. The skull grows in response to the enlarging brain. The *suture*, or growth, lines allow the skull to expand. The standard names of the major suture lines are: metopic (M, often functionally fused by the ninth month), sagittal (S), coronal (C), squamosal (SQ) and lambdoid (L). Coronal, metopic and sagittal sutures converge at the anterior fontanelle, the "soft spot," (AF). Note the posterior fontanelle (PF); it closes very early, often by four or five weeks of age. The major sutures become functionally fused once the brain stops growing, in the middle teens.

The bones of the skull vault are the frontal (f), parietal (p), temporal (t) and occipital (o).

episodes, new bone will be laid down at the suture lines, and the skull will become slightly larger than it otherwise would have been.

2. PHYSICAL CHARACTERISTICS OF THE SKULL AND INTRACRANIAL CONTENTS

The skull is a rigid, inelastic container for the brain. In technical terms, it has a "low modulus of elasticity;" it won't stretch or expand to accommodate sudden increases in intracranial volume. The shape of the skull calvarium, spheroidal, helps impart great resistance to compression and indentation.

Figure 2 is a midsagittal section of the skull with all contents removed. Note the "buttressing" effect along the skull base of the bony struts contributed by the sphenoid wings (sphenoid bone) and the petrous ridges (temporal bone). Only very great forces applied for relatively long periods of time are capable of deforming or crushing the skull base. Along the base, only the floor of the anterior fossa is thin and vulnerable; even here, considerable protection is provided by the thick orbital rims and the lateral orbital struts. The sturdy and wedge-shaped clivus — actually a part of the occipital bone — anchors the skull anteriorly and inferiorly. The sphenoid bone and the basal occipital bone contain the various foramina for egress of the cranial nerves from the skull. These foramina are extremely resistant to disruption. If this were not so, the relatively flimsy cranial nerves would suffer damage much more frequently during head trauma.

Note the course of the middle meningeal artery. Early in life, this artery lies imbedded in the dura, beneath the skull. As the skull thickens with age, the artery often comes to be incorporated into the bone particularly at the base of the skull. Fractures that cross the artery may lacerate it, allowing blood under high pressure to be pumped against the dura lining the brain. Such a blood clot, an extradural hematoma, may have dramatic consequences as we shall see later on (Figure 23).

Figure 3A shows a midsagittal view of skull and contents. Note that the brain literally floats in the skull cavity, cushioned by a layer of cerebrospinal fluid (CSF). One of the functions of the CSF is to act as a shock absorber for the brain. If the CSF were not there, the brain would slap against the skull with every movement of the head. This would happen because the skull and brain have different densities and masses. When the skull starts to move,

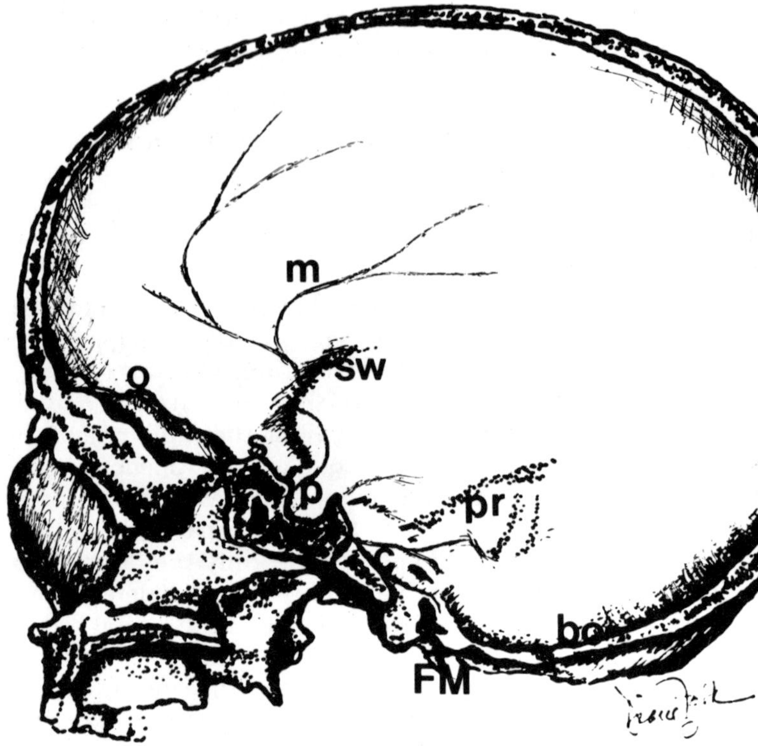

Figure 2. Skull, mid sagittal section.

The skull base is made up of the orbital plates of the frontal bones (o), the cribriform plates of the ethmoid bones (unmarked), the sphenoid bone (s) which houses the pituitary fossa (p), the clivus (c) which is a part of the occipital bone, and the basal occipital bone (bo). The foramen magnum (FM) is the hole in the basal occiput where the spinal cord is continuous with the medulla of the brain stem.

Sphenoid wing (sw) and petrous ridge (pr) are marked. Note the groove produced by the middle meningeal vessels (m).

the brain lags slightly because it is not firmly tethered to the skull anywhere. The CSF acts as a cushion at such times, as it does when the skull stops moving before the brain does.

Note that several of the surface cerebral veins cross from the brain to empty into large venous channels, the venous sinuses (Figure 3B). These bridging veins are vulnerable during times of rapid acceleration or deceleration of the skull, and they may tear, spilling venous blood out onto the brain surface (a subdural hematoma).

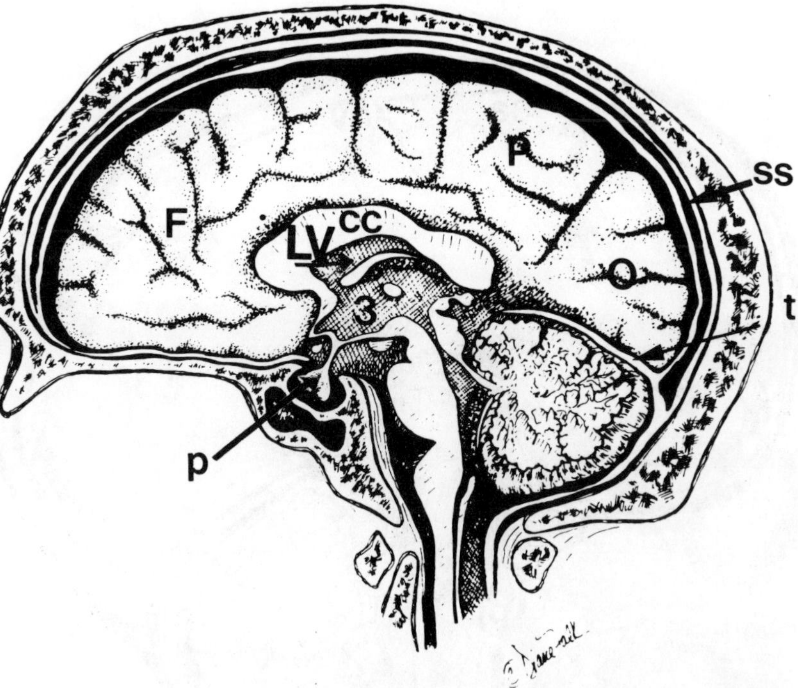

Figure 3A. Skull, mid sagittal section, with contents (semi-diagramatic). The brain floats within the skull cavity, cushioned by cerebrospinal fluid (CSF) in the subarachnoid space (here shaded black).

F — frontal	cc — corpus callosum
P — parietal lobe	t — tentorium
O — occipital lobe	ss — superior sagittal sinus
LV — lateral ventricle	p — pituitary gland
	3 — third ventricle

The brain is made up of a cellular parenchyma, walls of blood vessels, and perivascular and extracellular fluid-filled spaces. The parenchyma consists of *neurones*, the information processing and transmitting elements, and *glial cells* whose functions are complex — nutritive, supportive, reparative. Neurones are found in enormous numbers in the cerebral and cerebellar cortex and in collections deep in the brain, the various ganglia or nuclei. The outgoing and incoming processes of neurones are called axons and dendrites respectively. They often travel in bundles in the "white matter" of the brain, and these fibres are supported by glial cells. Glia exist in great numbers in the cortex and nuclei as well.

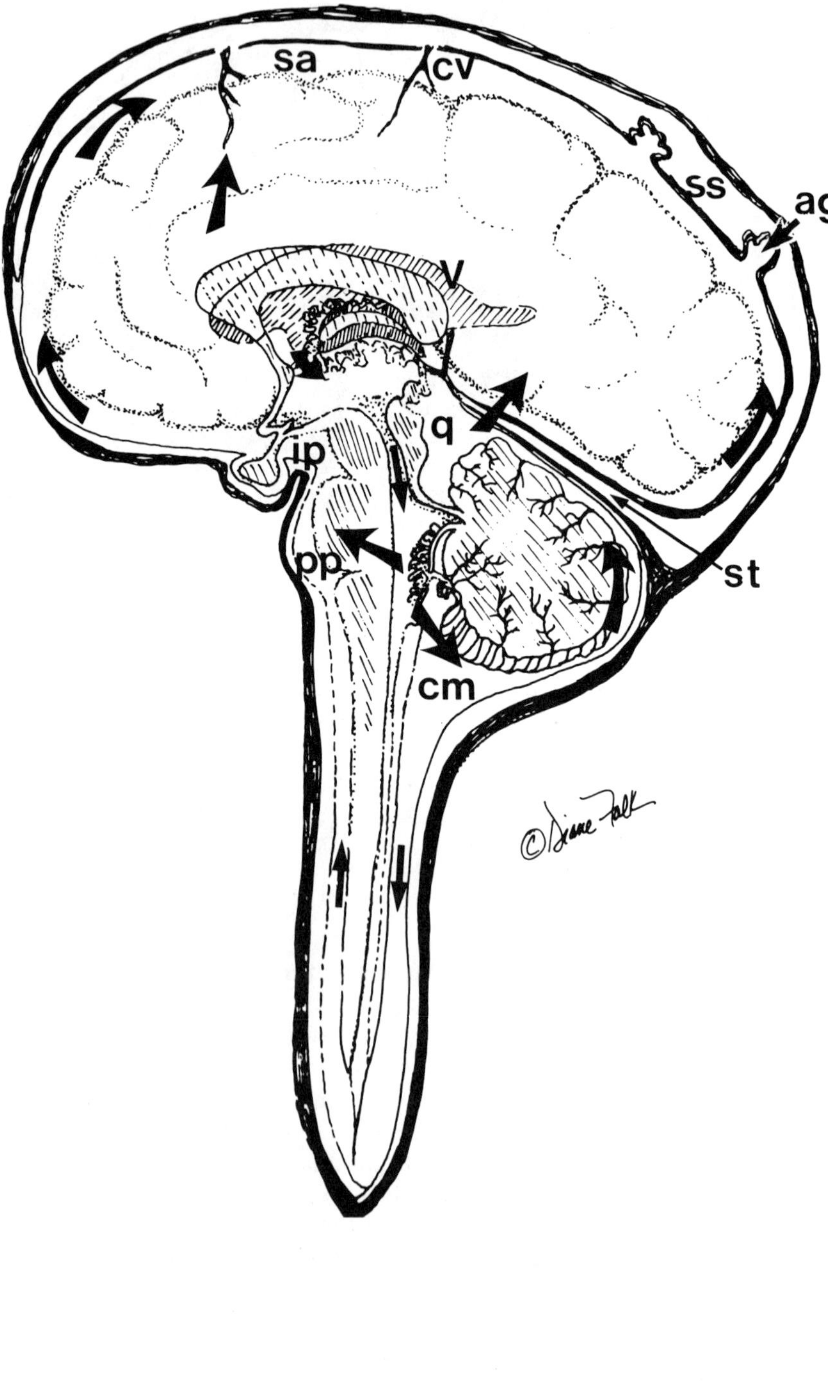
sa
cv
ss
ag
v
q
ip
pp
st
cm
©Diane Falk

Because of the water content of cells and the extracellular spaces, the brain acts more like a liquid when pressure is applied — it cannot be compressed. How important this fact is we shall see subsequently. Furthermore, the brain is *not* a homogenous gel. The felt-work intricacy of cortex and nuclei contrasts with the fibrous nature of white matter. Junctional zones between grey and white matter tend to be quite sharply demarcated. When the brain is suddenly set in motion, especially when rotational vectors are involved, shearing stresses occur between tissue layers, potentially with very serious results.

The intracranial cavity is divided partially into three compartments (Figure 4A). The *tentorium*, a double layer of inner dura reflected from the petrous ridges and the occipital bone, is shaped like a tent with its apex nearly at the central point of the skull cavity. It separates the *posterior fossa* from the *supra-tentorial compartment.* Anteriorly, in the midline, the edges of the tentorium diverge to form an elongated gap, the *incisural opening.* Another doubly-reflected layer of the inner dura, the *falx cerebri*, partially separates the supra-tentorial compartment into right and left *hemicalvaria.* Both the tentorium and the falx are tautly stretched, and their free edges are quite sharp and rigid. Posteriorly and inferiorly, the falx helps suspend the tentorium in the midline.

Figure 4B also indicates sites of potential danger for the brain whenever it is set violently in motion with respect to the skull. Even though the skull is lined by smooth dura, the floor of the anterior fossa is rather uneven. The inferior surface of the frontal lobe is easily bruised, even lacerated, when it moves rapidly over these bumps. The same damage may occur to the inferior temporal

←

Figure 3B. Sagittal section of skull and contents.

This illsutration shows an exaggerated subarachnoid space (sa), and a lateral ventricle (V) is drawn in. The arrows indicate the direction of flow of the CSF. Some of the cisterns are indicated:

q — cistern of quadrigeminal plate
cm — cisterna magna
pp — prepontine cistern
ip — interpeduncular cistern

Two arachnoid granulations (ag) are shown, protruding into the superior sagittal sinus (ss). The straight sinus (st) lies within the tentorium. Two cerebral veins are seen (cv), crossing the subarachnoid space to empty into the sinus.

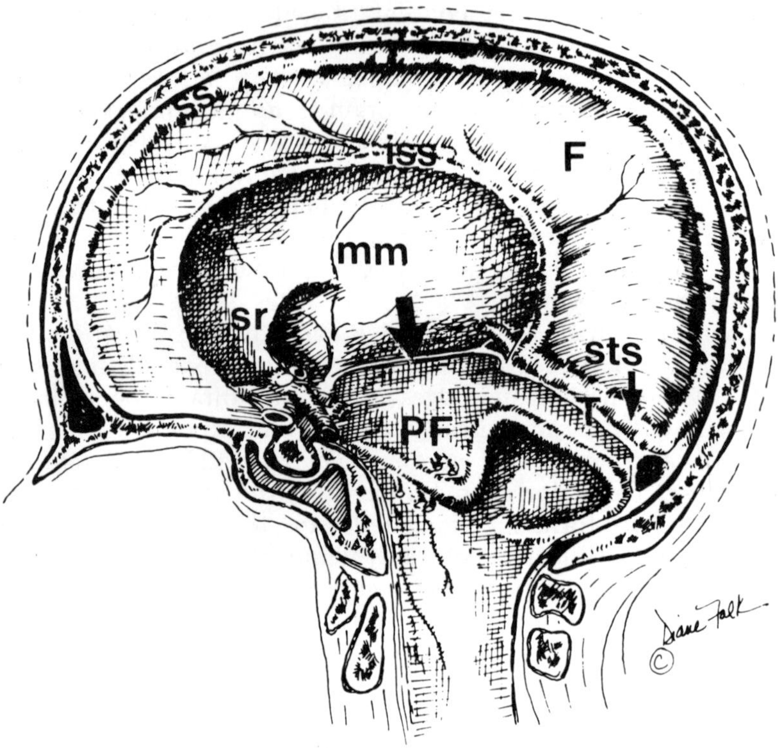

Figure 4A. The cranial compartments.

T — tentorium (cut edge)
F — falx
ss — sagittal sinus (superior)
sts — straight sinus
iss — inferior sagittal sinus
sr — sphenoid ridge
mm — bony grooves, middle meningeal artery
PF — posterior fossa

The heavy arrow marks edge of the incisural opening.

surface from abrasion along the petrous ridges. Brain laceration is a common result when the brain is pushed hard and relentlessly against the wing of the sphenoid bone, the edge of the tentorium, or the edge of the falx. Thus, the buttresses and the internal supporting structures of the skull may become instruments of damage during the brief moments of head trauma.

Where the layers of tentorium and falx diverge to join one another or the skull, potential cavities are formed. Nature in her wisdom has used these rather triangular spaces (*venous sinuses*) as conduits for venous blood to leave the brain. Figure 5 is an illus-

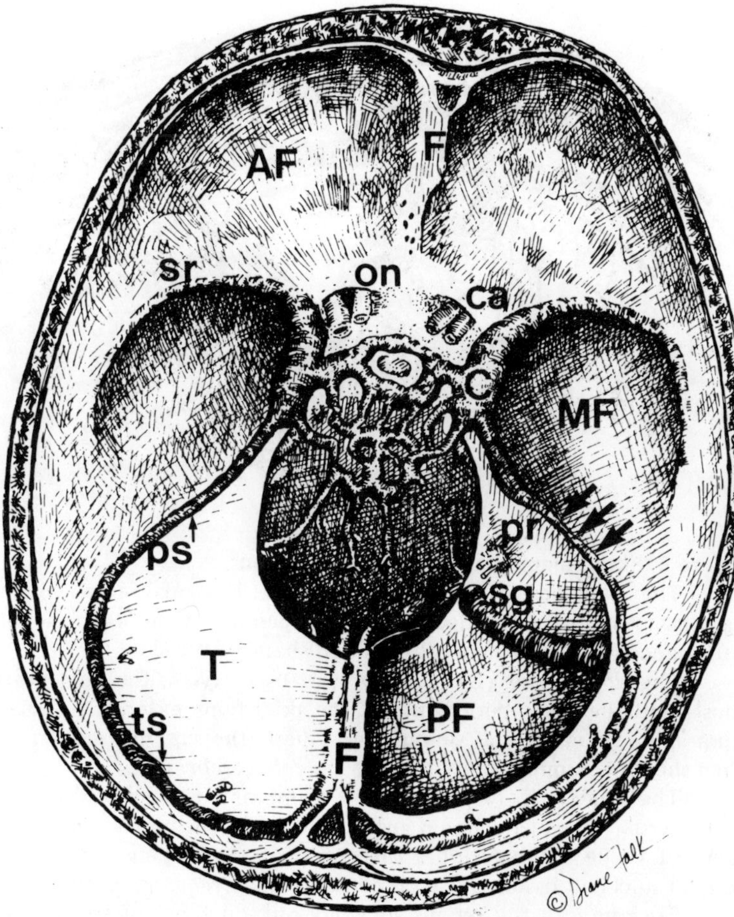

Figure 4B.

AF — floor of anterior fossa	MF — middle fossa
sr — sphenoid ridge	PF — posterior fossa
on — optic nerve	sg — sigmoid sinus
ca — carotid artery	T — tentorium
C — cavernous sinus	pr — petrous ridge
F — falx, cut edge	ps — petrosal sinus
ts — transverse sinus	

Anteriorly, the tentorium attaches along the apex of the petrous ridge (three small arrows). The anterior slope of the petrous ridge is in the middle fossa, the posterior slope is beneath the tentorium in the posterior fossa. Note that the tentorium on the right side has been cut away, allowing a view of the posterior fossa.

The superior sagittal sinus can be seen in the cut edges of the falx both anteriorly and posteriorly.

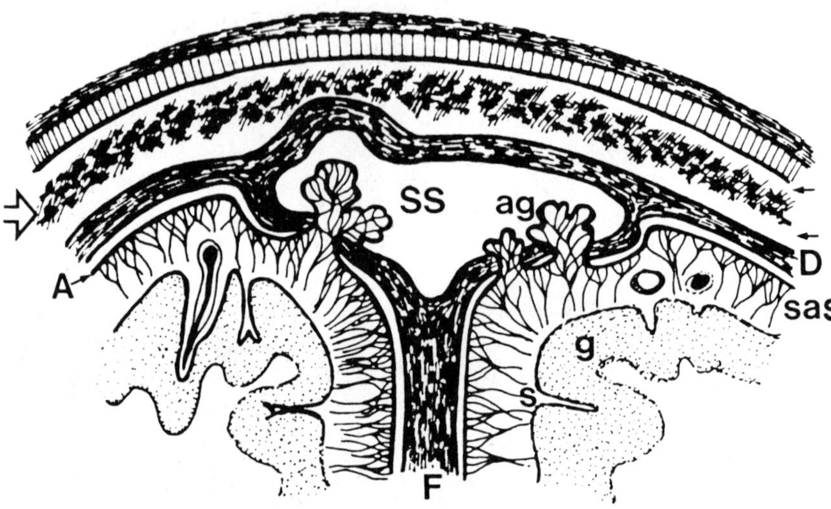

Figure 5. Skull, meninges, superior sagittal sinus.

The skull has a laminar construction. The small arrows point to the hard inner and outer cortical bone; the open arrow points to the intervening soft (cancellous) bone. Note the vaulted shape of the skull.

The *dura mater* (D) is really two fused layers: the dura proper innermost, and the inner periosteum of the skull lying externally. Note how the dura splits to enclose a venous sinus, here the *superior sagittal sinus* (SS), then the inner laminae unite to form the *falx cerebri* (F).

The *arachnoid* ("spider-like") membrane (A) gives off many septae which cross the subarachnoid space (sas) to reach the *pia mater*, a gossamer layer of tissue that envelopes the entire brain, hugging the cortical surface into all sulci and fissures. The sas contains the *cerebrospinal fluid*.

Sticking into the venous sinus are outpouchings of arachnoid cells, the *arachnoid granulations* (ag). These are covered by a layer of venous endothelial cells. Through the arachnoid granulations, the bulk of the cerebrospinal fluid is reabsorbed into the blood stream.

The folds of brain surface are called gyri (g), and the valleys between are sulci (s).

tration of this arrangement. Because the walls of venous sinuses are thick and tough, and because of their triangular shape, it is virtually impossible to occlude a large venous sinus by pressure alone. Cerebral veins, in contrast, are thin-walled and are easily compressed and collapsed.

The skull has a laminar construction (Figure 5). The inner and outer lamina are hard, cortical bone, whereas the middle diploic layer is soft, vascular, cancellous bone. This laminated structure, along with the vaulted shape, gives the skull extraordinary strength considering its thickness. Nevertheless, because bone has little or no elastic property, the skull is brittle and liable to fracture in circumstances that we shall discuss later.

The brain is covered by three layers of tissue, the *meninges* (Figure 5). The *dura mater* is tough and fibrous. It consists of two laminae, the outer one being the inner periosteal layer of the skull. The dura lines the skull internally. The *arachnoid* is next, and between dura and arachnoid is the potential *subdural space.* The arachnoid loosely envelopes the brain, here and there jumping across from prominence to prominence of brain surface and thereby creating large cavities or *cisterns* (Figures 3B and 11). Intimately covering the brain is the *pia,* a gossamer layer of cells that invests every nook and cranny of the brain surface. Between the arachnoid and pia is the subarachnoid space, which contains the cerebrospinal fluid (CSF). The CSF is found, as well, within the *ventricles* of the brain (Figures 3B and 7). The ventricles are cavities in which CSF is produced and from which the CSF flows to cover the surface of brain and spinal cord. There are four ventricles, a lateral ventricle in each cerebral hemisphere, the third ventricle between the hemispheres, and the fourth ventricle in the midline in the posterior fossa. Ventricles communicate with one another by the *foramina of Monroe* (lateral and third), the *aqueduct of Sylvius* (third and fourth), and with the subarachnoid space via the *foramina of Luschka and Magendie* of the fourth ventricle.

Note how the brain surface is folded into complex patterns of *gyri* (the brain cortex) and *sulci* (the pia-lined spaces between gyri). This arrangement allows much more surface area to be packed into the same volume. It is the surface cortex of the brain that contains the complex neuronal groupings that produce our consciousness and our intellectual and motor abilities. Very deep sulci are called *fissures.* Several of the gyri and fissures are regular features of the brain surface, and have been assigned standardized names (Figure 6). Similar functions tend to be grouped together in certain areas of the cortex, but that discussion is reserved for Chapter 3.

In general, the large arteries which carry blood into the head lie on the brain surface (Figures 7 and 10B). Distribution branches leave the parent artery, usually at right angles, to penetrate the brain parenchyma. At various levels, but particularly in or near

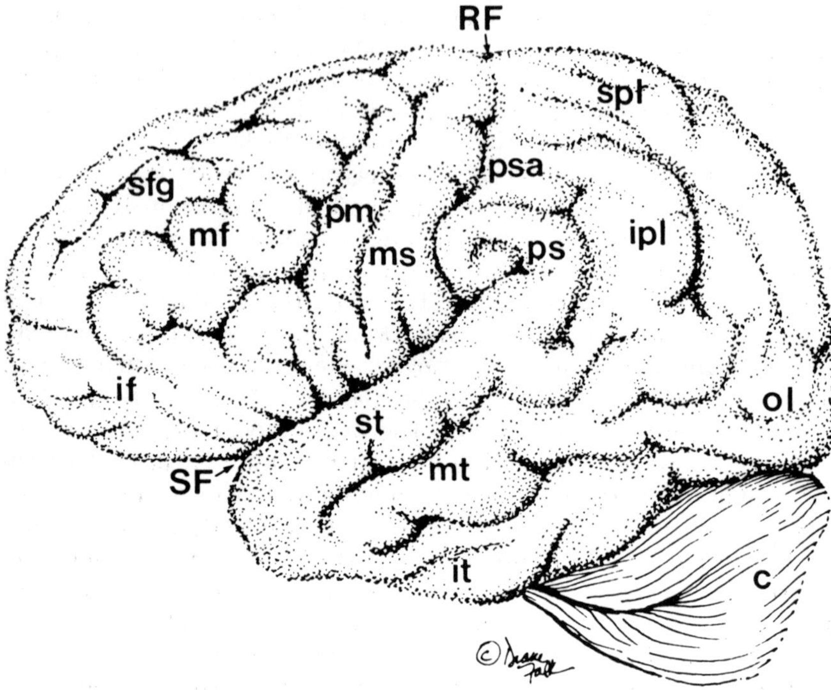

Figure 6. The lateral brain surface.

FRONTAL LOBE
sfg — superior frontal gyrus
mf — middle frontal gyrus
if — inferior frontal gyrus
pm — premotor area
ms — motor strip

PARIETAL LOBE
psa — primary sensory area
spl — superior parietal lobule
ipl — inferior parietal lobule
ps — parasylvian gyrus

TEMPORAL LOBE
st — superior temporal gyrus
mt — middle temporal gyrus
it — inferior temporal gyrus

OCCIPITAL LOBE — ol

CEREBELLUM — c

FISSURES
SF — Sylvian fissure, hiding the *insula*, marks frontal lobe above and temporal lobe below. The over-foldings of the brain that cover the insula (Figure 7) are called *opercula.*
RF — Rolandic fissure, separates frontal lobe anteriorly from parietal lobe posteriorly.
Note how large the frontal lobe is, compared to the others.

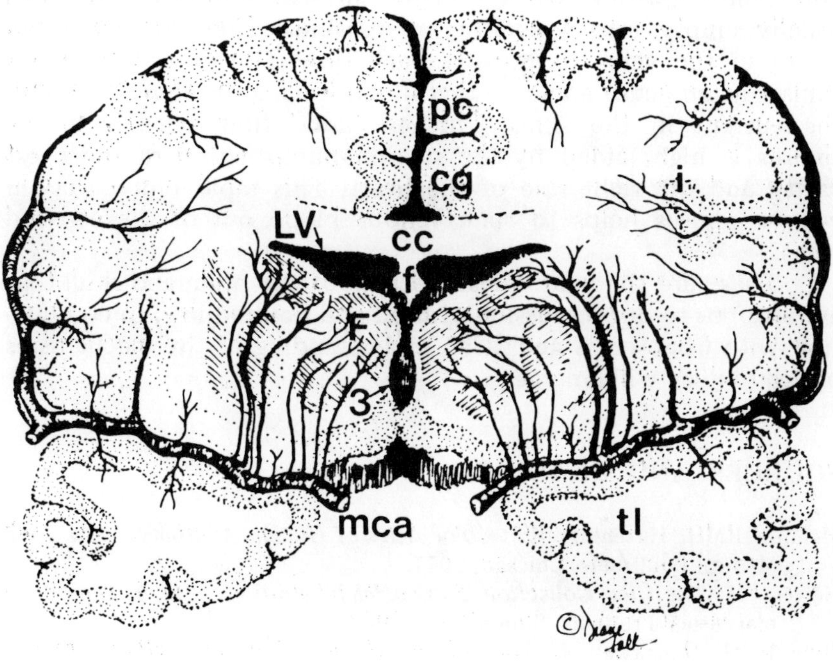

Figure 7. A coronal section of brain.

NAMED STRUCTURES

cc — corpus callosum, carrying nerve fibres from one hemisphere to the other, allowing analagous cortical areas to communicate.

cg — cingulate gyrus

pc — para-cingulate gyrus

i — insula

f — fornix, communication pathways from medial temporal lobes to medial thalamic nuclei

LV — lateral ventricle

3 — third ventricle

F — foramen of Monroe

tl — temporal lobe

mca — middle cerebral artery. Note how penetrating arteries leave parent trunk at right angles, entering brain substance. There are tiny anastamoses between the end-vessels of adjacent arteries.

grey matter, the small nutritive branches leave, dividing several times, finally ending in the capillary plexuses where nutritive and gas exchange occurs with brain tissue. The veins that collect the blood beyond the capillary plexuses tend to follow the course of companion arteries. Once on the surface, however, the veins usually empty into a nearby venous sinus. There are no reflux valves in the veins to prevent back flow. However, veins enter sinuses at an acute angle, so that blood leaving the vein flows with the current in the sinus. Further, blood flow velocity in the sinuses is high, aided by the suction-pump action of the chest cavity and the right side of the heart. This rapid blood flow in venous sinuses helps to suck venous blood out of the cerebral veins.

These are the anatomical features of the brain and skull that are apropos to our discussion of head and brain injury. In conjunction with Chapters 3 and 4, an understanding of the mechanisms of head injury will emerge.

SOURCES AND READINGS

McMinn RMH, Hutchings RT: *Color Atlas of Human Anatomy.* Year Book Medical Publishers, Chicago, 1977.

Netter FH: *The Ciba Collection of Medical Illustrations.* Vol. 1. Ciba Pharmaceutical Products, Summit, NJ, 1953.

Roberts M, Hannaway J: *Atlas of the Human Brain in Section.* Lea and Febiger, Philadelphia, 1970.

CHAPTER 3

Physiology

1. CEREBRAL METABOLISM THE HIGH COST OF ENERGY

Neurones are the most specialized cells in the body, and among the most vulnerable to many types of insult. Simply, the neurone is concerned exclusively with the processing and transmission of information, from periphery to brain, from one area of brain to another, from brain to periphery. The brain is the "soul" of the body; by it we live and move and have our being. The death of the brain now is widely recognized as signalling the end of individual human existence even though other organ systems may carry on normal function.

Most neurones are small, gathering information from nearby cells, processing it, and modulating the responses and activities of other nearby cells. But some neurones are the largest cells in the body. For example, a so-called pyramidal neurone of the motor cortex may have a process (axon) that travels all the way to the lower terminal of the spinal cord, a distance of nearly a meter in tall individuals. The metabolic requirements of such a cell are prodigious.

Neurones communicate with one another by means of *synapses.* Figure 8 depicts a typical small neurone and the sites of synaptic contacts. The cell body alone of a neurone may be covered with tens of thousands of synapses. Most synapses on the dendritic tree are excitatory to the cell, while synapses near the outlet of the axon tend to be inhibitory. Almost all synapses function by transmission of a chemical activator across the synaptic cleft from incoming axon to receiving dendrite or cell body. These transmittor chemicals are manufactured in the cell body of the neurone, passed down the processes, and perhaps further refined

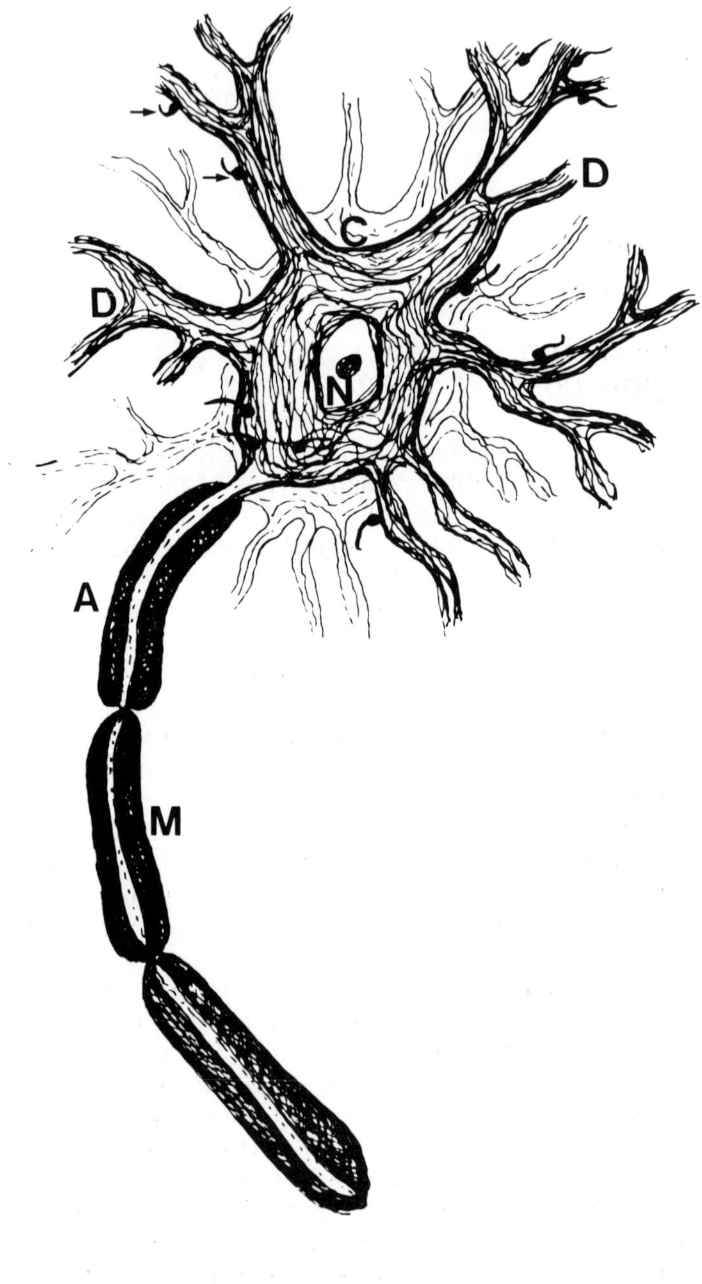
D
C
D
N
A
M

in the pre-synaptic terminal. There is a reverse flow of fluid from the axon terminals to the cell body, but the composition and function of this current is not well understood.

Information travels along cell processes and over the cell body by means of a wave of change of trans-membrane electrical potential. A complex interaction of ions of sodium, potassium, chlorine, hydrogen and perhaps bicarbonate is maintained by so-called membrane pumps. Electrical polarization of the neuronal membrane depends upon precise ion concentrations on each side of the membrane, and the membrane pumps are responsible for reconstituting these ionic gradients.

The upshot of all of this is that enormous quantities of energy are consumed by neurones. The principal factories of such energy are the *mitochondria*, subcellular organelles whose special and only function is the conversion of the energy substrates glucose and oxygen into compounds that release energy on demand in other parts of the cell.

During the long development of the nervous system, neurones have given up a very important function in order to

←

Figure 8. A neurone.

This cell is the information processing and transmission unit for the nervous system. The *cell body* (C) is filled with cytoplasm and innumerable small organelles. Within the *nucleus* (N), all of the cell's DNA resides, directing the metabolic and other functions of the RNA of the cytoplasm. The dendrites (D) convey incoming information toward the cell body, and the single axon (A), covered by its thick *myelin* (M) envelopes, carries the cell's integrated and modulated output to the periphery or to another neurone.

Information is passed from cell to cell by *synapses*, marked by small arrows. Because the dendritic tree has a huge surface area, the majority of synapses occur on dendrites, usually onto a small spike protruding from the dendrite, a *spine*. Depending upon the physical and chemical properties of the synaptic junction, the synapse may be inhibitory or excitatory to the receiving neurone.

Most synapses contain acetylcholine as the transmission chemical. When a critical amount of transmittor impinges upon the receiving membrane, an electrochemical "depolarization" of the membrane occurs. This electrical change travels along the dendritic membrane like a wave, and if sufficiently strong, the entire neurone responds by initiating a current flow down the axon. The myelin sheath of the axon allows the current to skip along the fibre at great velocities, up to 120 meters per second in some human neurones.

specialize in information processing and transfer: they are able to store only small amounts of energy substrate. For practical purposes, the brain is dependent upon a steady and sufficient supply of glucose and oxygen delivered by the blood stream. If the supply of either substrate is interrupted for more than a few minutes, neurones will die. Glucose cannot be converted efficiently to high-energy compounds if oxygen is not supplied freely, and oxygen — a very active and toxic chemical — cannot be detoxified adequately within the cell if there is insufficient glucose to supply the great metabolic demands of the mitochondria.

For these reasons there exists a crucial symbiotic relationship between brain metabolism and neuronal function, and cerebral blood flow.

2. CEREBRAL BLOOD FLOW THE VITAL PIPELINE

Apart from the heart muscle, the brain requires a higher percentage per weight of the cardiac output than does any other organ. Yet the volume of blood in the brain at any one instant is not very large: only 50 to 75 ml. Of great importance to the brain is the fact that cerebral blood flow (CBF) remains virtually constant over a wide range of mean systemic arterial pressures (MAP). Figure 9 illustrates this cerebral blood flow curve. Note that between mean systemic arterial pressures of about 40 to 160, CBF increases only slightly.

This trick is accomplished by an automatic reflex on the part of small arterioles in the brain, a reflex termed *autoregulation.* Autoregulation of CBF is essential for bipedal creatures; otherwise we would faint every time we stood up. At the high end of the curve, a MAP over 160 or more "breaks through" the autoregulation, and CBF rises in a linear fashion with blood pressure. Such high pressures in small cerebral arteries or arterioles may cause a catastrophic hemorrhage, such as is seen in hypertensive crises. Below MAP of 40 or so, CBF falls off very rapidly. A good clinical example of such a situation is shock from blood loss. A person in severe shock for a prolonged interval may sustain brain damage because of significantly reduced cerebral blood flow.

Between the blood vessels and the brain parenchyma there exists a "blood-brain barrier" (BBB). This barrier is made up, probably, of the basement membrane of the tiny blood vessels, the

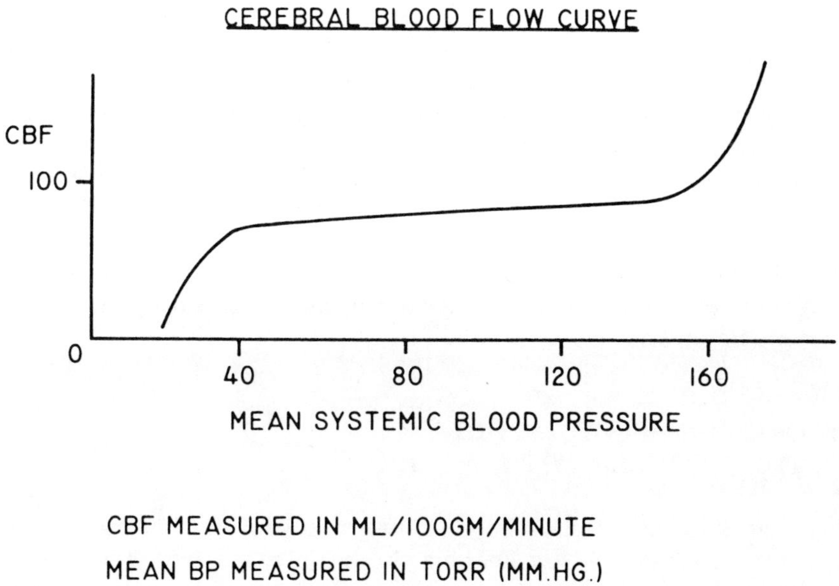

Figure 9. The relationship between cerebral blood flow and mean systemic blood pressure.

The "autoregulation" reflex in the cerebrovascular capacitance vessels — pre-capillary arterioles, capillaries, post-capillary venules — ensures that CBF remains virtually constant over a significant range of systemic arterial blood pressure.

CBF is but one component of oxygen supply to the brain. Neurones must be able to extract oxygen and glucose from blood. *Oxygen uptake* may be impaired in any inflammatory or infectious condition of the brain, by cerebral edema, by neuronal poisoning, to name a few factors. *Oxygen availability* to the neurone may be compromised by severe anemia, ischemia or vascular occlusions, severe hypocapnia and carbon monoxide poisoning — where a normal concentration of oxygen in the blood is too tightly bound to the hemoglobin molecule to be extracted by the cells, and by hypoxemia.

The neurone's demand for oxygen can be reduced by drugs such as barbiturates and by physical conditions such as hypothermia. In such circumstances, the brain may tolerate a substantial reduction in CBF without ill effect.

very tight junctions between individual endothelial cells of these vessels, and a transport function of endothelial cells termed pinocytosis. Certain compounds normally are totally excluded from the brain, others are admitted freely. It seems that lipid composition, certain stereo configurations of chemical bonds, and size and degree of molecular hydration, are some of the determining factors in the selectivity of the BBB.

The important point here is that the BBB can be disrupted, usually with deleterious effects upon the brain. Hypoxia, ischemia, toxic chemicals, hyperosmolar solutions, and trauma are factors thay may induce breakdown in the BBB. Regions of brain where the BBB is inactive usually swell and lose function. Within the small blood vessels in such regions, autoregulation usually is defective as well, and unregulated blood flow through these vessels may add to the local problems, sometimes in the form of catastrophic hemorrhage.

3. CEREBROSPINAL FLUID THE TROUBLE WITH WATER

We have seen how the CSF helps to protect the brain by a cushioning effect and by keeping the brain suspended in a watery medium. The CSF is an actively secreted, specialized fluid that looks like water. Its composition resembles that of plasma except for a much lower protein content. There are approximately 150 ml in the ventricles and the entire subarachnoid space of the brain and spinal cord at any one time. Some 70 percent of CSF is actively produced by the *choroid plexuses* of the ventricles. The rest of the CSF is added in the ventricles and subarachnoid spaces as fluid entering from perivascular spaces. The latter component may be termed "brain water," and it contains end-products of cerebral metabolism and activity.

As long as blood flows through the choroid plexus, CSF will be formed. The rate of CSF production is approxiamtely 0.35 ml per minute. In the course of any one day, we produce about 500 ml of CSF. Since the normal head and spinal canal contain only 150 ml of CSF at any one time, obviously there is a turn over of CSF about every eight hours. This fact implies that CSF circulates and is absorbed somewhere (Figure 3B).

CSF is produced in all four ventricles; because most of the choroid plexus is in the lateral ventricles, most of the CSF is formed there. Then by bulk flow, the CSF moves through the ventricular system and enters the subarachnoid space of the posterior fossa. The CSF circulates rather sluggishly over the brain surface, most of it eventually being absorbed back into the blood stream through small outpouchings of arachnoid that stick into the venous sinuses, particularly the superior sagittal sinus along the midline at the top of the skull. The important point is that CSF absorption is a passive process, while CSF production is an active process. Normally, you absorb as much CSF as you produce, over the course of a day.

The principal cause of trouble with the CSF and brain water inside the head is: there is no feed-back system to control the rate of production of CSF. Only when pressure within the head gets so high that blood can no longer enter the skull does production of CSF cease. We shall discuss the consequences of this fact in Chapter 4. The system is poorly designed from the standpoint of a hydraulic engineer.

The CSF has functions other than shock absorption. Certain drugs and chemicals placed into the CSF are able to penetrate directly into the brain, principally through the lining membrane of the ventricles, the ependyma. This and other evidence suggests that CSF may have a nutritive function for subependymal and subpial cells.

Within the third ventricle, the CSF has been shown to carry certain hormonal precursors (especially gonadotrophic) from posterior areas of the hypothalamus to nuclei near the eminence of the pituitary stalk. Thus, the CSF has a transport function.

Because most of the CSF is actively secreted, and because the CSF has a well-defined flow pattern, the actively produced CSF serves as a diluting liquid for brain water. The latter may contain rather toxic end-products of cerebral metabolism and chemical activity. In this manner, CSF acts as a "sink" for brain water.

Finally, in situations where intracranial pressure (ICP) is rising rapidly, the fact that some CSF usually can be expelled from the head means that the CSF system may act as a "buffer mechanism" for ICP.

4. REGIONAL LOCALIZATION IN THE BRAIN

The mapping of functional areas of the cerebral cortex and of certain deep nuclei of the human brain has been accomplished largely during operations under local anesthesia to remove epileptogenic foci, during stereotactic procedures on the deep nuclei — usually done to control movement disorders, or during investiga-

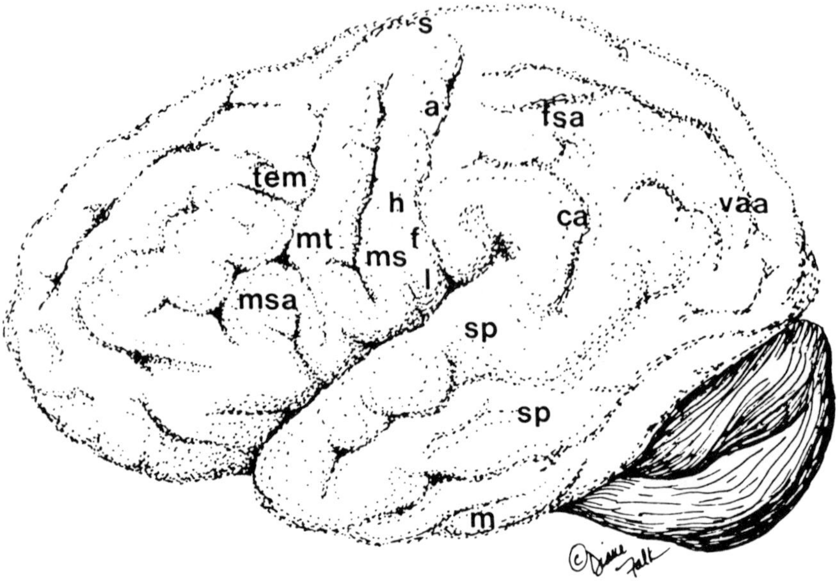
s
a
fsa
tem
h
ca
vaa
mt
f
ms
l
msa
sp
sp
m
©Diane Falk

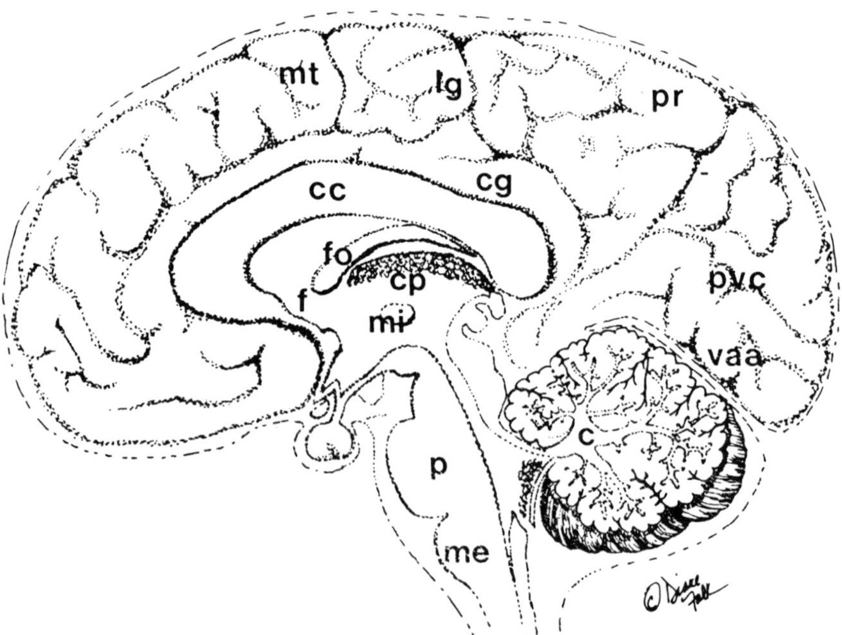
mt
lg
pr
cc
cg
fo
cp
f
mi
pvc
vaa
c
p
me
©Diane Falk

Figure 10A. Cortical localization.

This illustration shows the lateral surface of the left cerebral hemisphere and the medial surface of the right. Figures 6 and 7 may be referred to for cortical area designations. General localizations are given.

FRONTAL LOBE: These large structures have much to do with the nebulous entities of intellectual content, social inhibitions, judgment, behavior. Specific functions include:

- msa — motor speech area (Broca's convolution)
- tem — tracking eye movements
- mt — muscle tone and readiness
- ms — fine motor activities, for lips (l), face (f), hand (h), arm (a), shoulder (s), leg (lg)

PARIETAL LOBE: Inferiorly, overlap occurs into the temporal lobe. The "non-dominant" parietal lobe plays a major role in interpretive, perhaps emotional, functions. Some refer to it as the "artistic" lobe.

- fsa — fine sensory appreciation, body image
- ca — symbolic language interpretation, calculation
- pr — pattern recognition, spacial constructs.

TEMPORAL LOBE

- sp — speech. In general, more posterior areas have to do with the interpretation of auditory and visual speech, more anterior areas with motor functions.
- m — memory. The entire brain takes part in permanent memory storage. Medial and inferior temporal lobes appear to house the mechanisms for sorting and processing of recent memory experiences.

OCCIPITAL LOBE

- vaa — visual association areas
- pvc — primary visual cortex

NAMED STRUCTURES

- cc — corpus callosum
- f — foramen of Monroe
- cp — choroid plexus in roof of third ventricle (3)
- mi — massa intermedia, a band of glial tissue uniting the medial thalami, traversing the third ventricle
- fo — fornix
- c — cerebellum
- p — pons
- me — medulla
- cg — cingulate gyrus

tion of epileptic patients who have had electrodes placed in deep nuclear structures. Animal work has been of particular benefit with respect to the humoral and vegetative functions of the hypothalamus and brain stem nuclei.

Figure 10 indicates the major functional areas of the cerebral cortex. During head trauma, specific damage may be done to restricted cortical areas by such things as indriven skull fragments, perforating objects, or by small localized hemorrhages. More diffuse surface and deep white matter injury often results from dramatic acceleration/deceleration head movement, particularly when a rotary component is involved.

The medial temporal lobes have a special importance in regards to memory. The consensus is that bilateral medial temporal lobe injury is almost certain to interfere seriously with the acquisition or recall of new memories. Even so-called "trivial" concussions, with periods of loss of consciousness for only moments, may interfere with a child's ability to assimilate new information for periods of up to six weeks.

We once heard statements such as: "We only use 10 percent of our brain, anyway." Such opinions arose from lack of knowledge about cortical function, and many areas of the brain were assumed to be "silent." Neuropsychology has made tremendous advances during the past decade, and the neuropsychologists' success in investigating and clarifying regional brain function have been most helpful to medical clinicians. It is seen now that all cortical areas function in a closely integrated fashion and that no cortical area is silent or permanently in reserve. The terms "dominant" and "non-dominant" now must be qualified as to precise functions. The left temporal and parietal lobes may be "dominant" for speech, but the analagous areas of the right hemisphere have a crucial interpretive, perhaps creative function that makes language richer for many people. The so-called "non-dominant" hemisphere certainly has come into its own in the past few years.

Young children have a plasticity of cortical function that is largely lost with age. For example, a surface laceration of the speech centers of the left hemisphere probably will not prevent a child of less than two or three years from acquiring normal speech and comprehension of language. Probably the analagous cortical area of the right hemisphere assumes that role. But even in mature adults, astounding recoveries of function sometimes occur. A well-known actress has managed an amazing recovery of her speech following a large hemorrhage into her dominant (for speech)

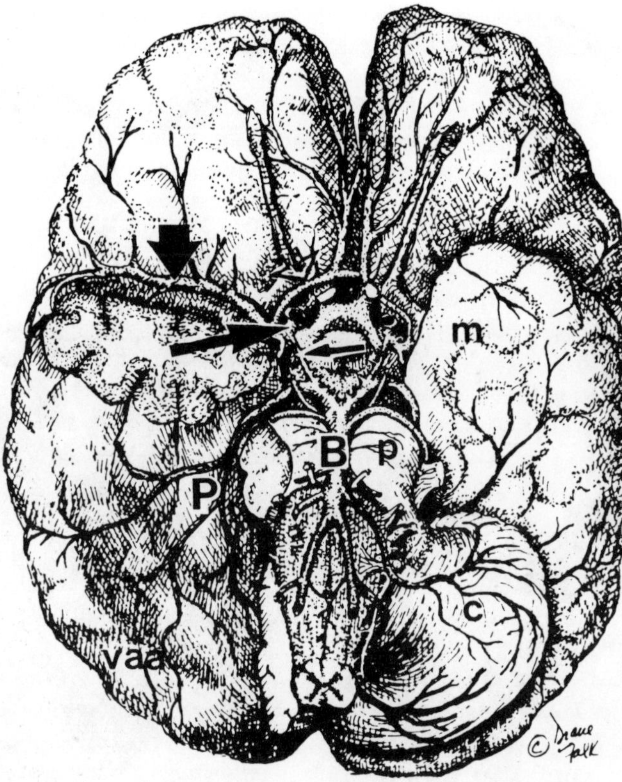

Figure 10B. Cortical localization, cerebral arteries.

This is an illustration of the undersurface of the brain, and of the major arterial supply to the brain. The key is the same as given for Figure 10A.

Note the *vertebral arteries* uniting to form the short, vitally important *basilar artery* (B), which then divides in the interpeduncular fossa into the *posterior cerebral arteries.* Small channels (*posterior communicating arteries,* small arrow) join the pca's to the *internal carotid artery* (long arrow). The anterior cerebral arteries (open arrow) unite across the midline via the *anterior communicating artery.* This network of vessels is called the *Circle of Willis.* The middle cerebral artery (heavy arrow) arises from the bifurcation of the internal carotid artery.

Violent motion of the brain within the skull often leads to bruising of the temporal lobe tips and the tips and under surfaces of the frontal lobes. Such damage may be reflected by memory deficits and social and judgmental abnormalities.

The *posterior cerebral artery* (P) and its branches irrigate the under surface of the occipital and temporal lobes. If the medial surface of the temporal lobe is forced medially (Figures 21, 22), this artery may become occluded, leading to infarction of these areas.

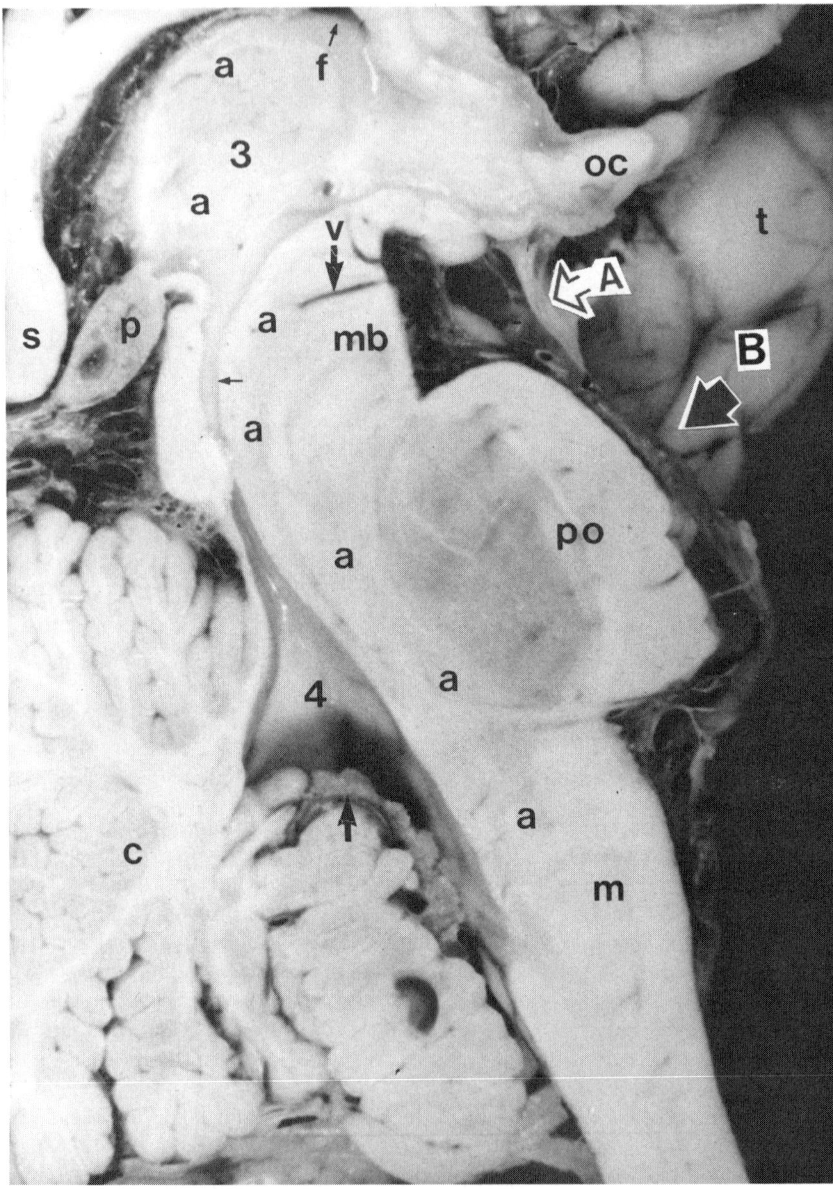

Figure 11. Midsagittal section of the brain stem.

a — extent of the various nuclei and fibre tracts that make up the *ascending reticular activating system* (see text).

A — open arrow indicates fold of the arachnoid that leaps across from the under-surface of the hypothalamus to front of pons. The space so created is termed a *cistern*, in this case the interpeduncular cistern.

B — heavy arrow points to basilar artery. From this vessel, midline perforating arteries enter the pons and midbrain (see text). The basilar artery arises at the lower edge of the pons at the junction of the two vertebral arteries, and ends by bifurcating into the two posterior cerebral arteries in the interpeduncular cistern.

C — cerebellum. Note the frond-like structure of the cerebellum. This large brain lobe sits in the posterior fossa behind the brain stem. It receives incoming impulses from position sensors in joints and muscles, via the spinal cord, and descending motor impulses from the cerebral cortex and brain stem motor nuclei. The output of the cerebellum is crucial for the control of motor activity throughout the body.

f — small arrow points to the foramen of Monroe, through which the lateral and third ventricles communicate.

m — medulla. This compact part of the brain stem carries all ascending sensory and descending motor pathways from and to the periphery. Some of its nuclei are intimately concerned with the control of cardiac and respiratory activity.

mb — midbrain. The nuclei of the third cranial nerve lie just anterior to the aqueduct of Sylvius (small arrow). These nuclei, and the nerves that emanate from them, control the size of the pupil of the eye. If either the nucleus or the nerve is damaged, the pupil will dilate. As an indicator of scale, the aqueduct normally is about 1 mm in diameter.

oc — optic chiasm. Here, the *optic nerves* join medially. Some of the optic nerve fibres — from the inner half of the retina — cross into the other *optic tract* in the chiasm.

po — basal part of the pons.

p — pineal gland. This enigmatic gland lies behind the third ventricle, in the subarachnoid space. Just behind and above it is the . . .

s — splenium of the corpus callosum, the most posterior part of that great cerebral commissure. Through the splenium, crossing fibres connect the visual areas of the brain.

t — temporal lobe, tip.

v — perforating midline artery into brain stem. Others are clearly visible in the basal pons.

3 — third ventricle. Note the bird's head appearance, the aqueduct of Sylvius forming the neck. The dark structure above and behind the roof of the ventricle is one of the deep cerebral veins.

4 — fourth ventricle. Note that the floor of the fourth is the posterior surface of pons and medulla. The tented roof of the fourth is the cerebellum. The lobulated structure on the lower roof of the fourth is choroid plexus (vertical arrow).

temporal lobe. Interesting phenomena are often documented, such as retention of singing fluency (perhaps a "non-dominant" temporal lobe function), or better preservation of a native language as compared to secondarily acquired ones.

Figure 11 is a sagittal view of the brain stem to indicate the areas of the brain responsible for the conscious state. This extensive and rather nebulous structure is often referred to as the *ascending reticular activating system* (ARAS). The exquisite clinical-pathological correlative studies of Plum and Posner have added greatly to our understanding of this vital structure.

This area of the brain stem is very vulnerable to direct and secondary injury as outlined in Chapter 4. It appears that the ARAS of the medulla and pons and lower midbrain functions principally to initiate and direct the conscious state, while the ARAS of the high midbrain, the subthalamus and thalamus acts largely to maintain alertness and attention. Certainly, destruction of the lower ARAS induces unremitting coma, whereas restricted lesions in the upper ARAS leave a patient in an altered conscious state but rousable to a higher one.

The ARAS receives enormous numbers of incoming sensory signals from the periphery, particularly the face and special sense organs. So environmental stimuli are integrated into the conscious state, with some therapeutic implications. For example, it is useful on occasion to have a radio playing softly at the bedside of a restless, stuporous patient, or a recording of voices of parents and siblings. The caveat is that patients who seem unlikely to form memories of events or conversations occasionally may recall snippets of what has gone on around them. The lower ARAS also has a major role in the regulation of that physiological state of coma, sleep.

You will perceive from Figure 11 that small hemorrhages or infarcts in this nebulous structure may have devastating effects. Even with the rest of the brain intact, a small blood clot in the pontine ARAS may condemn the head injury victim to endless coma.

SOURCES AND READINGS

Amacher AL, Delmaestro RF: Nutrition, volumes, ions, and radicals. In: *Pediatric Neurosurgery. Surgery of the Developing Nervous System.*

Shulman K, and McLaurin RL (Eds.). Grune and Stratton, New York, 1982. Chapter 64.

Davison H: *Physiology of the Cerebrospinal Fluid.* Churchill, London, 1967.

Fishman RA: *Cerebrospinal Fluid in Diseases of the Nervous System.* WB Saunders Co., Philadelphia, London, Toronto, 1967.

Kandel ER, Schwartz JH: *Principles of Neural Science.* Elsevier/North-Holland, New york, Amsterdam, Oxford, 1981.

CHAPTER 4

Pathophysiology. Why things go wrong.

1. MECHANISMS OF HEAD INJURY

For all practical purposes, there must be relative motion between the skull and the brain for concussion or brain damage to occur during head trauma. The principal exception is with perforating injuries of the skull. It makes little difference whether the head strikes upon or is struck by another object, and brain injury may occur even without head impact when sudden acceleration/deceleration forces are applied. For example, serious damage can be done to the brain surface, with tearing of surface veins and production of an acute subdural hematoma, by violent shaking of an infant if the babe's head is unsupported. However, the overwhelming majority of head injuries involve head impact of some description.

The effect of head impact upon the brain depends upon several factors. Some of these are: the magnitude of the force applied; the intracranial vectors of transmitted force; the time of contact between head and object; the thickness of scalp and skull; the region of the skull that bears the brunt of the impact; whether or not the skull fractures. Figure 12 is an illustration of such factors.

Obviously, the greater the force applied to set skull and brain in motion, the greater the potential damage — other things being equal. But any and all events that occur superficially will reduce the amount of force available to produce brain injury. For instance: it is commonly found that a patient who has sustained a large scalp laceration, a fractured skull beneath the cut, perhaps even a laceration of dura and superficial brain tissue, enters the

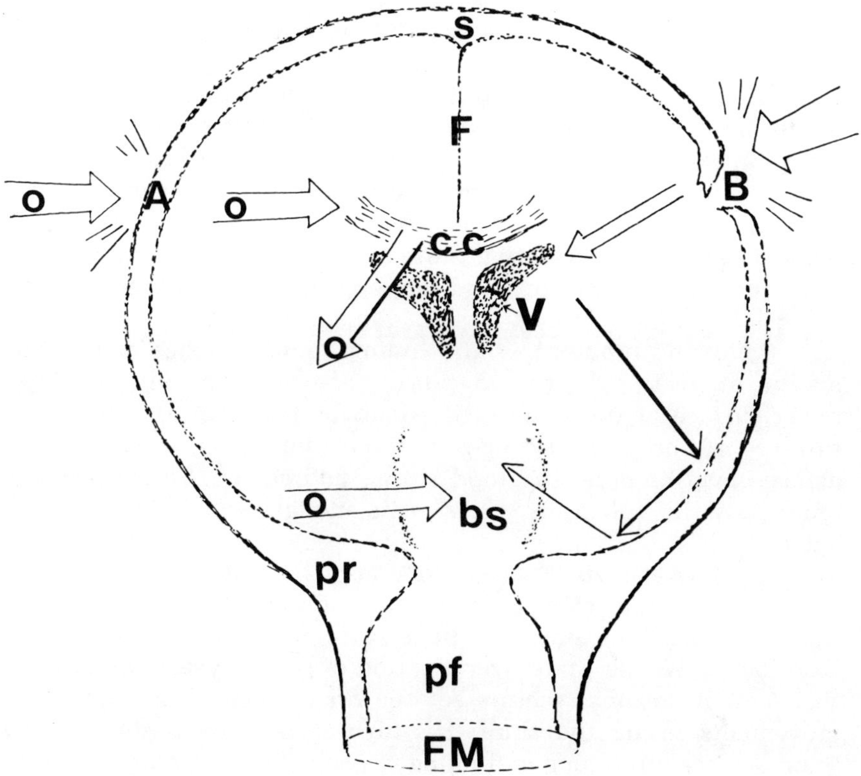

Figure 12. Coronal section of skull and contents, diagrammatic.

s — skull
pr — petrous ridge
pf — posterior fossa
F — falx
cc — corpus callosum
V — lateral ventricle
FM — foramen magnum
bs — brain stem, upper

An impact at A that does not cause a skull fracture allows virtually all of the force of impact to be transmitted into the head. The force vectors will reflect from such surfaces as the falx, ventricular wall, midline structures (arrows marked o), eventually concentrating in the upper brain stem.

At B, the impact has caused the skull to fracture, dissipating much of the force, which may be further attenuated by a dampening effect provided by fluid in small quantities leaving the ventricle.

emergency room awake and talking. Superficial structures have absorbed most of the force of the blow and the deeper brain centers are spared.

At the moment of impact, the brain begins to move relative to the skull. The brain may slap against the skull directly beneath the point of contact, then rebound. Because the brain is not a homogenous gel, small cavities may form for microseconds at the junction between cortex and white matter (Figure 13). Small blood vessels may tear during those episodes, causing small cortical and subcortical contusions and hemorrhages. If such lesions occur extensively, a great deal of cortical damage may result.

Following rebound of the brain, similar damage may occur on the opposite side, the so-called "contre-coup" injury. If the under surface of the brain rattles back and forth across the rough surfaces of the petrous ridges or the orbital roofs, severe surface damage may be done to blood vessels and cortex. Sometimes the brain hits the sphenoid wings with enough velocity to lacerate itself.

As dramatic as these events may be, much more serious injury may ensue when a rotational component is introduced to the brain-skull movement. The elegant and epochal studies of Gurdjian at Wayne State over a period of several years emphasized this fact. Rotational vectors set the brain to swirling and gliding movements inside the skull. His high-speed movies showed the brain surface stretching and piling up, veins tearing, blood pouring out onto the brain surface, even an occasional artery ripping and pumping out blood under high pressure. I recall wondering how the human organism could survive even a vigorous head shaking!

Such shearing forces eventually become concentrated in the brain stem. The skull has only one foramen large enough to allow for the escape of significant kinetic energy, the foramen magnum. Energy entering the skull must be dissipated in some fashion. Either it escapes or it is absorbed by the skull contents; it cannot magically disappear.

You will appreciate from Figures 3 through 14 that the cerebrum and brain stem resemble a mushroom. When the heavy cerebral hemispheres begin to move — rotate, especially — relative to the brain stem, gray and white matter damage frequently ensue. Sabina Strich, a British neuropathologist, showed that brains that had sustained traumatic injuries years before showed clear-cut evidence of the events. Shearing injuries in the deep white matter of the hemispheres and in the brain stem were extremely common.

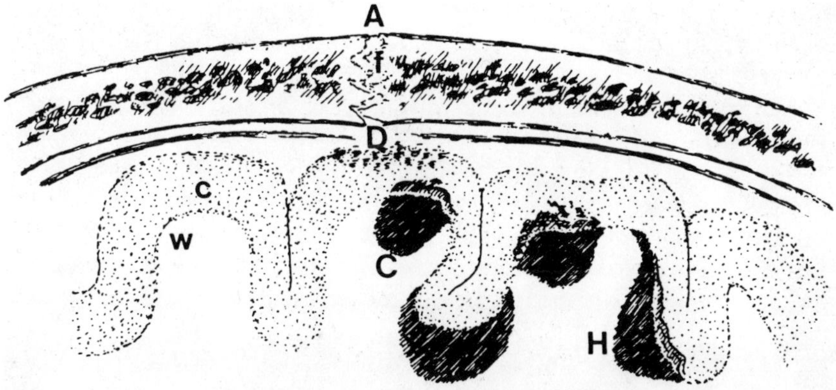

Figure 13. Subcortical effects of an overlying impact.

An impact at A has caused a fracture (f), with direct bruising of the cortex and laceration of the dura at D. The brain surface is depressed, then it rebounds. There may be a lag in motion between the cortex (c) and white matter (w), causing small cavities (C) to form for a few milliseconds. Small blood vessels tear, and blood flows into these areas, producing deep cortical and subcortical hematomas (H). These hematomas usually are very small and multiple.

Axons of cells located in the cerebral cortex were disrupted deep in the brain; those cells' output had been lost forever. The disturbing thing was that such damage was seen even after "trivial" head injuries. Of course, the clinical evidence has been before us for decades; the "punch-drunk syndrome" is nothing more than the cumulative effects of many "minor" head injuries. Figure 14 emphasizes the vulnerability of the brain stem when the cerebrum is set into violent motion.

The brain may be injured in other ways, as well. A simple linear skull fracture may, at the moment of depression of the bone edges, lacerate the brain. In-driven bone fragments, pieces of clothing, or perforating objects damage brain directly.

A special case exists for gunshot wounds, particularly for rifled shells. The radial velocity of these projectiles imparts a tangential destructive force to the brain, and the track of brain destruction is much wider than the diameter of the bullet. Figure 15 is a dramatic illustration of such an injury. The track of carnage fills up with brain debris and blood. Absorption of certain chemicals liberated from smashed brain may induce a systemic consump-

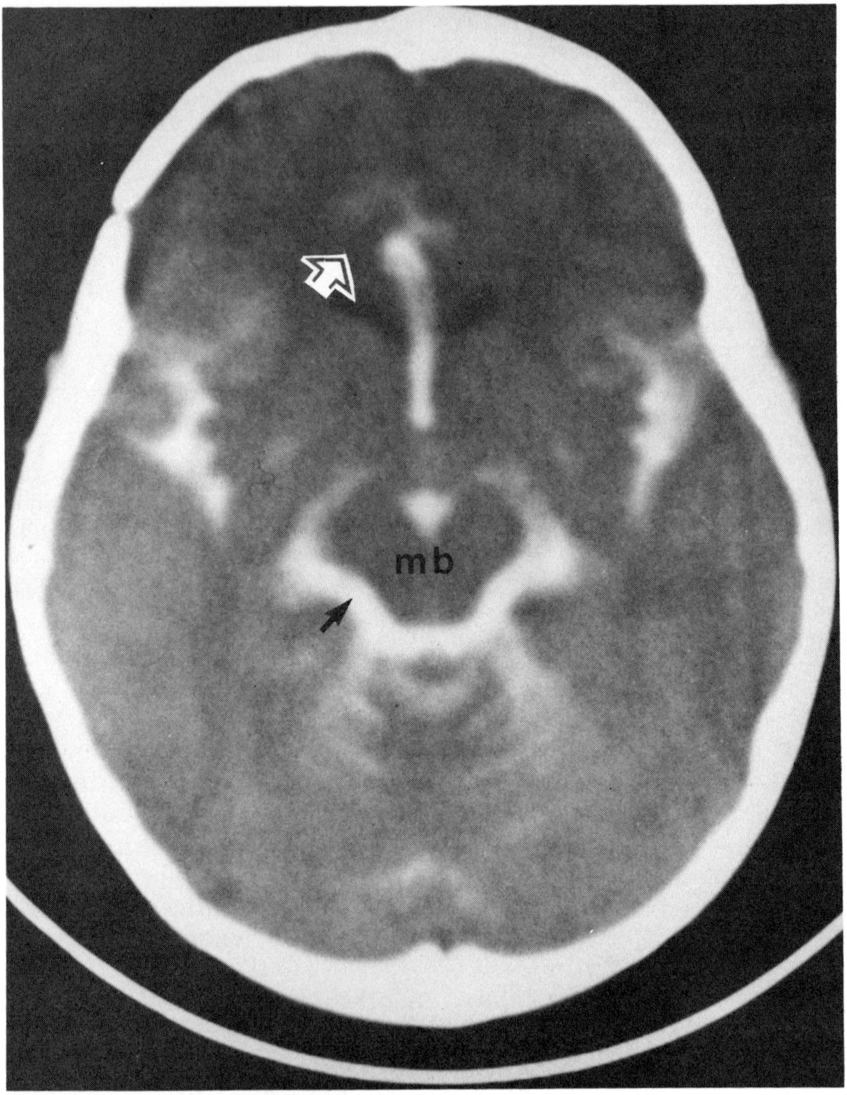

Figure 14. Horizontal (half-axial) CT scan cut of the brain.

Some of the subarachnoid space cisterns are filled with a water-soluble contrast material (dark arrow). The open arrow points to the frontal horn of the lateral ventricle.

The midbrain (mb) is well-outlined by contrast. Note how centrally located the midbrain is. It is the "stem of the mushroom." Imagine the rotational shearing forces that may concentrate here when the brain above is set into violent, swirling motion.

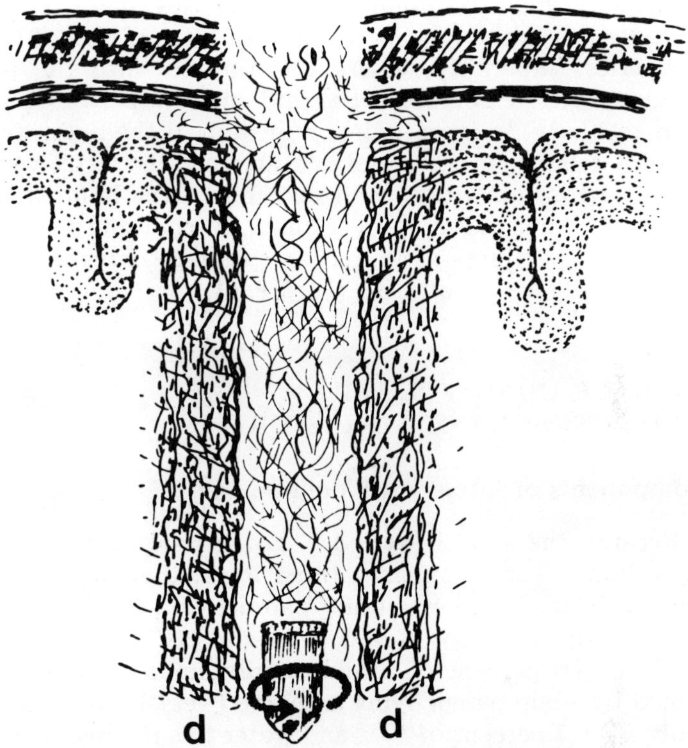

Figure 15. A gunshot wound of the brain.

Rifled projectiles rotate at great velocities, producing destructive forces that extend perpendicular to the path of the bullet. Here, the skull has been perforated. The bullet tears out its own track, which becomes filled with blood and smashed brain. Some of this debris escapes the head through the entry wound, some spills onto the brain surface. Bone fragments, hair and bits of anything worn on the head will be found in the track.

There is a zone of brain destruction (d) surrounding the bullet track, where the radial forces generated by the bullet have pulverized the brain.

tion of blood-clotting elements leading to a condition known as a *coagulopathy.* It is suspected that certain prostaglandins are of major importance in such events.

In subsequent sections, we shall see how secondary effects of brain injury complicate the problem. But first, examine Figures 7, 10B and 11 once again. Note how the major arteries ride on the brain surface, in the subarachnoid space, and how their branches usually perforate brain tissue at right angles. The basilar artery is a particularly good example for our purposes. It is "tethered" at both ends: inferiorly, as it is formed by the junction of the vertebral arteries; superiorly, where it bifurcates into the posterior cerebral arteries. Circumferential and midline perforating vessels leave it regularly, to irrigate the brain stem. If the brain stem is set in motion relative to its supplying arteries, the latter very easily may be torn, often within the substance of the brain stem. Such brain stem hemorrhages, even if small, disrupt and destroy brain stem nuclei and fibre-tracts that are passing through. The consequences usually are devastating (Figure 24).

2. INTRACRANIAL VOLUME AND INTRACRANIAL PRESSURE

a. Components of Intracranial Volume

Because the skull is, at most ages, a rigid container, it has a fixed volume. There are only three items that normally belong inside the head. These are: brain parenchyma and walls of blood vessels; blood; water, both brain water and CSF.

About 70 percent of available intracranial volume (ICV) is occupied by brain parenchyma and blood vessel walls. Blood takes up only 5 to 7 percent of ICV, and water fills the rest. Most of the water is in the perivascular and extracellular spaces, a smaller volume in the ventricles and subarachnoid spaces.

It is useful to think about ICV in this way, as we shall see later in this chapter. Figure 16 is a representation of the components of intracranial volume.

b. The Meaning of Intracranial Pressure

When a needle is introduced into the cerebrospinal fluid in the spinal arachnoid space of an individual, as may be done for diagnostic purposes, a pressure value can be recorded. In a quiet person, lying on the side with head and torso on the same level, the cerebrospinal fluid pressure usually will be about 120 mm of water, or 8 to 9 mm of mercury (torr). In such a situation, the CSF pressure may be considered to represent intracranial pressure (ICP).

The measurement of ICP requires a reference point, the right atrium of the heart. The reason for this is that the filling volume

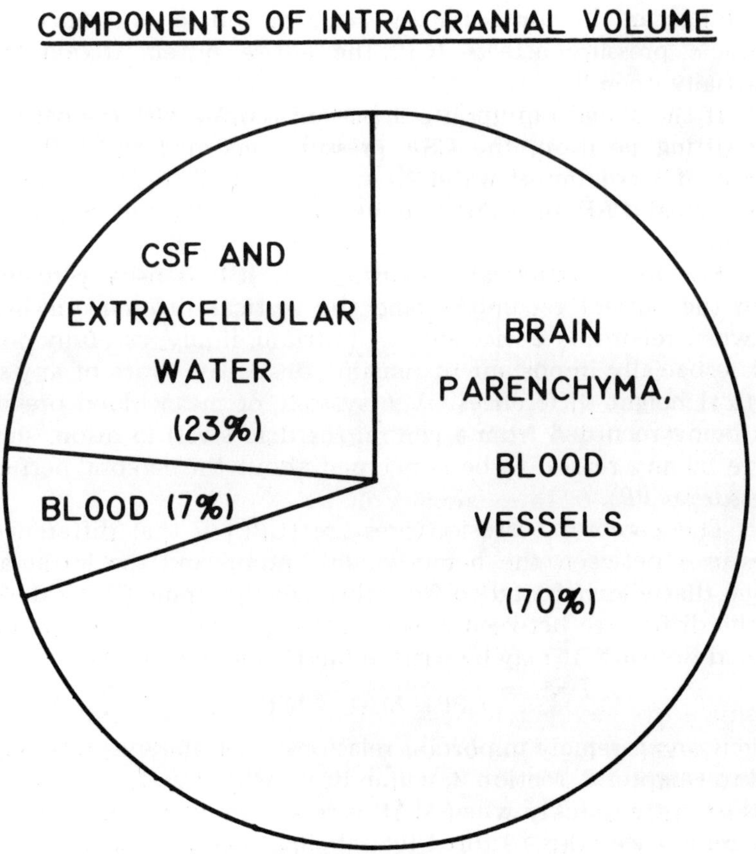

Figure 16. Components of intracranial volume.

When intracranial volume (ICV) is increasing quickly, only some 30% of normal ICV is available as a "buffer"; in practical terms, the buffering capacity might be 25% of buffer volume, or about 7 to 8% of ICV. A typical adult ICV might be 1400 ml. Thus, an abnormal volume of 100 ml very well might exceed intracranial buffering capacity, in an acute situation.

Extracellular water includes the fluid between cells and in the perivascular spaces. CSF includes the ventricular and subarachnoid space volumes.

and pressure of the right heart determine the volume of blood that may leave the head in any unit of time. Pressure in the thorax changes constantly in a cyclic fashion because of the expansion and contraction of the chest wall; for example, during spontaneous inspiration intrathoracic pressure falls. The cyclic alteration in intrathoracic pressure affects right atrial pressure, as well. Since the lungs are in contact with the atmosphere, and since intrathoracic pressure affects ICP, the entire system is said to be "partially open."

If the spinal tap upon our patient is done with the patient in the sitting position, the CSF pressure recorded will reflect the height of a column of water from top of skull to the needle. The intracranial CSF pressure will be negative relative to the right atrium.

For many practical reasons, then, ICP is usually recorded with the patient recumbent and the vertical difference in height between recording device and right atrium, if any, carefully noted. It is especially important to remain constantly aware of any such vertical height differences when systolic or mean blood pressures are being recorded from a central (cardiac level) location, should there be any reason to be concerned about the cerebral perfusion pressure (CPP).

The cerebral perfusion pressure (CPP) is that difference in pressures between the hemodynamic pump and the intracranial space that allows blood to flow through the brain. CPP is defined as the difference between mean arterial pressure (MAP) and intracranial pressure. It may be written (and remembered) as:

$$CPP = MAP - ICP$$

This is an extremely important relationship. Reference to Figure 9 and to Chapter 3, section 2, will indicate why. Cerebral blood flow falls off very quickly when MAP is less than 40 mg Hg (torr). For this reason we take 40 torr CPP as being the critical lower limit of safety; in injured brains, this lower limit well may be higher.

When recording ICP on a strip of paper, certain constant components of the wave form are seen (Figure 17). At fast recording speeds, two features emerge. The wave form marked by the long arrow is a ballistic wave due to the cardiac cycle. The upstroke represents the integrated systolic surge in the cerebral blood vessels. The downstroke represents the diastolic cycle; the notch frequently seen on this side of the wave is caused by a venous backwash from the emptying contraction of the right heart. Normally, the ICP pulse pressure (the height of the ballistic wave upstroke) is only 2 or 3 torr.

The cycle marked by the horizontal arrows on Figure 17 indicates the respiratory contribution to the ICP wave forms. Note that the ICP pulse pressure (ICPpp) increases somewhat at the top of the wave. The ebb and swell of blood leaving the head, with a

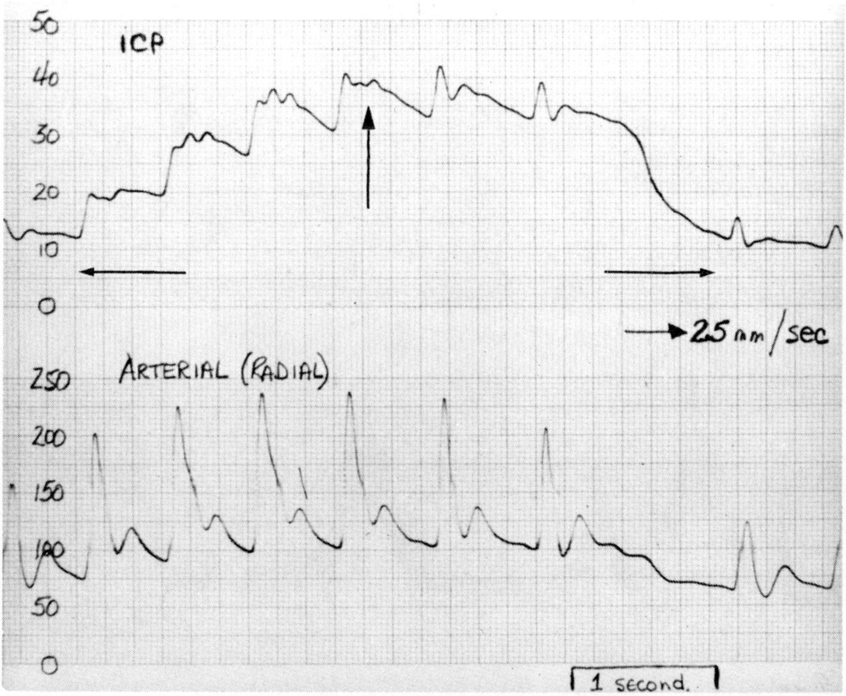

Figure 17. Components of the intracranial pressure wave.

ICP is recorded on the top strip, arterial blood pressure from the radial artery on the lower strip. The paper speed is 25 mm per second. Pressure readings are in torr (mm Hg). For details, see text.

virtually constant input on the arterial side, causes this small variation in ICP. The ICPpp increases because the brain is a little stiffer (less compliant) when venous volume is at its maximum.

Abnormal changes in ICP are best appreciated at slow paper speed. The designations given to these pathological waves in the earlier ICP literature are best forgotten. The point of overriding importance is that ICP waves that reduce CPP below critical levels for more than a few seconds are very dangerous, and may have a cumulative effect. Sometimes such increases in ICP occur very quickly, sometimes much more slowly (Figure 18).

c. The Relationship Between ICV and ICP

Following head injury, any factor that leads to an increase in ICV will cause a rise in ICP. The increment in ICV may come from

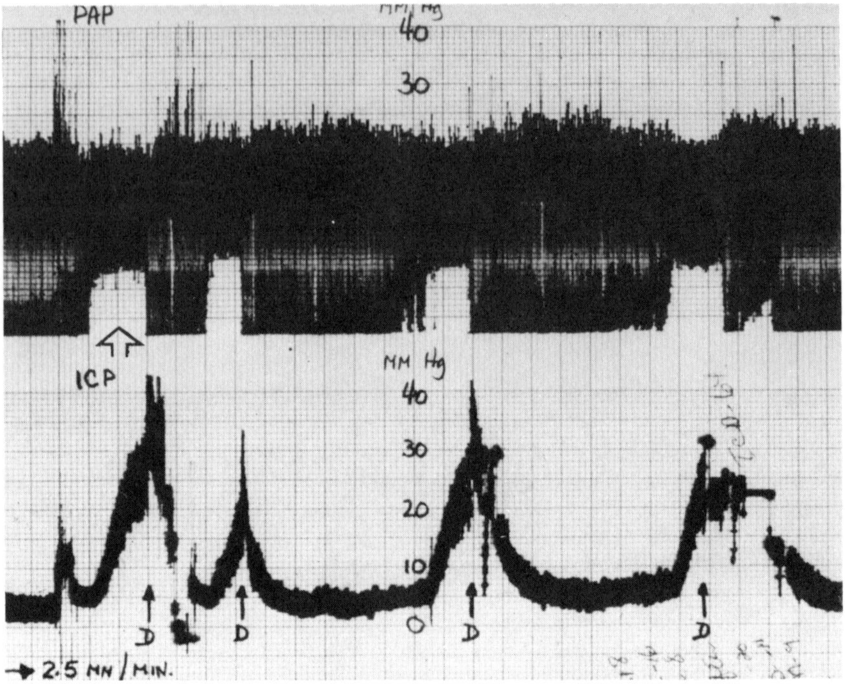

Figure 18. A clinical ICP recording.

The upper tracing is of pulmonary artery pressure, recorded from a Swan-Ganz catheter. The lower record is ICP. Paper speed is 2.5 mm per minute, so each large square represents two minutes real time. Pressure recordings are in torr (mm Hg).

This patient was in controlled ventilation per endotracheal tube and pressure-controlled respirator. Note the ICP waves, onsetting rapidly and peaking at 40 or more torr systolic pulse. "D" marks the event of opening the ventricular catheter to a drainage bag, to control ICP by volume drainage.

The sudden elevations in pulmonary artery diastolic pressure (open arrow) that occur in some patients at the onset of an ICP wave, are well demonstrated in this patient. When they are present, they indicate that a major ICP rise is imminent.

any one of, or any combination of, the components of intracranial volume, or from the formation of a collection of blood, fluid or pus not normally found inside the head. For practical purposes, when considering a rapidly changing physical situation within the skull, ICV and ICP are virtually interchangeable terms. To reduce ICP quickly, one must reduce ICV. There are ways of doing so, as we shall see shortly. Figure 19 demonstrates the critical relationship between ICP and ICV.

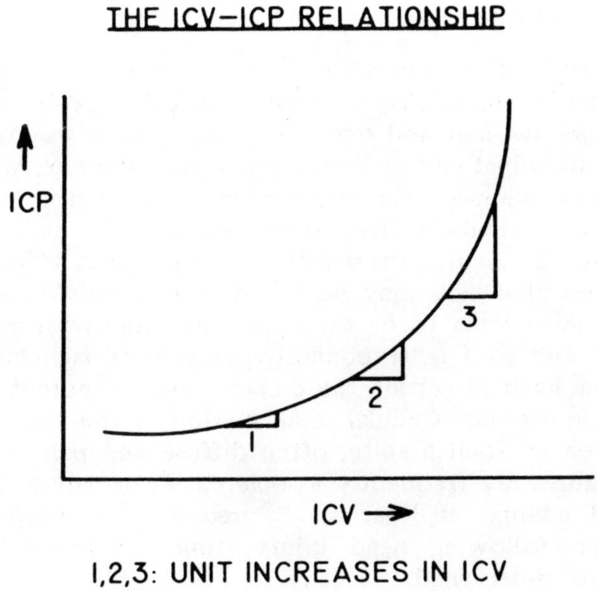

Figure 19. The ICV-ICP relationship.

See text. At event number 1, a unit increase in ICV elicits a small rise in ICP. On this part of the curve, the buffering capacity intracranially is substantial.

A patient on the curve at event number 2 is in more danger, as the ICP rise induced by a unit volume increase is greater. In technical terms, the intracranial *compliance* is falling. Compliance is measured as change in volume divided by change in pressure, or $\Delta V/\Delta P$.

At event number 3, intracranial compliance has fallen even further. A patient on the curve at this point is in very serious danger. If the induced ICP increase compromises cerebral perfusion pressure, sudden and catastrophic neurological deterioration may occur.

3. CEREBRAL SWELLING AND CEREBRAL EDEMA

These terms often are used interchangeably, though to many of us they have slightly different connotations. Both terms imply an increased water volume in the skull. Probably it is safest to use only the term "cerebral edema," with a qualifying phrase to indicate where the increased water load is. But very often the types of cerebral edema described below meld into one another. Nevertheless, it is useful to classify cerebral edema as follows.

a. Cytotoxic Edema

Here, the cells are overloaded with water, the extracellular and perivascular spaces may be compressed. At operation, such a brain appears swollen and dry, amd may have a woody consistency. The principal culprit here is the cell membrane. Membrane pumps cannot maintain the micro-environment within and without the cell. Particularly the sodium leak into the cell, down its concentration gradient, carries with it a large water volume. Both neurones and glial cells may be affected. One would expect the causes to such edema to be those that interfere with membrane physiology, and so it is. Hypoxia, hypoglycemia, ischemia, membrane toxins such as certain toxic chemicals, are potent inducers of cytotoxic edema. Cellular malfunction is the usual clinical manifestation of such a state, often diffuse and pan-encephalopathic. Seizures are frequently associated. Fortunately, this type of cerebral edema, at least as a predominant component, is seldom seen following head injury, unless cerebral hypoxia/ ischemia have supervened.

b. Vasogenic Edema

If the mean arterial pressure (MAP) is excessively high, or if vascular wall integrity has been compromised by local injury or inflammation, vasogenic edema may occur. Basically, this is a hydrostatic-force edema, with more fluid than usual being driven out of blood vessels into the extravascular and extracellular spaces. The fluid resembles plasma but with a lesser protein content, and it may contain a few red and white blood cells. The extracellular-intracellular osmotic gradient usually is not altered significantly, though some intracellular water accumulation may occur if the process persists.

Early on, the effects of vasogenic edema principally are those of locally raised tissue pressures. If the local pressure effects become excessive, however, the small arterioles and capillaries in the area may collapse, producing local ischemia. Further, local diffusion of oxygen to nearby cells may be reduced, as molecular oxygen normally does not diffuse more than about 150 microns from its vessel of origin. Thus, vasogenic edema may induce a secondary cytotoxic edema. This form of cerebral edema is very common following severe brain injury.

If one performs a CT scan on a patient with cerebral edema, the affected tissue has a less than normal density because of the increased water volume present. There is an entity much feared by pediatric neurosurgeons, the so-called "post-traumatic malignant cerebral edema." I have watched it onset after apparently trivial head bumps, destroying a child in a matter of hours. It seemed to be an intractible mystery until it was recognized during CT scanning of such children that the cerebral swelling noted was *hyper*dense, not *hypo*dense. This fact meant that the brains of such children were being excessively perfused with blood, hence the abnormal hyperdensity. Immediate control of respiration and therapeutic hyperventilation in such situations would reverse the process and prevent the evolution of the dreaded malignant cerebral edema. The entire situation was an example of an erroneous assumption on the part of clinicians, an error that could be rectified only when a suitable diagnostic imaging technique became available.

c. Interstitial Edema

Here, excess water lies in the intercellular spaces, principally in the white matter. Very little is known about this type of cerebral edema, and it is seldom associated with head injury. In any situation, it seems to be quite benign.

4. INTRACRANIAL "BUFFER" MECHANISMS FOR ICV AND ICP

Just as we speak of chemical buffer systems that help regulate the acid-base balance of the blood or of the urine, we may discuss physical buffer systems that help regulate ICV, hence ICP.

The term "buffer system" implies the dampening or moderating of a chemical or physical change that otherwise would occur too rapidly or that would exceed tolerable limits. We have discussed the components of ICV. Unfortunately, brain parenchyma makes up 70 percent of ICV, and the only way to reduce brain volume is to remove some of it. In most situations this is undesirable. Mind you, if the tip of a temporal or frontal lobe has been smashed beyond all hope of any cellular recovery, its removal may be recommended. But cortical and white matter bruising is usually widespread following severe head trauma, and the surgeon's instinct should be to conserve as much potentially functional brain as possible. For several reasons, craniotomy for removal of brain tissue following trauma is done less commonly now than it once was. One major reason is that we are better at manipulating the other components of ICV.

a. Intracranial Blood Volume (IBV)

Without doubt, the cerebral veins act as a reduceable reservoir of blood in many situations. They collapse easily, blood runs off through nearby veins that do not collapse. Sometimes, local brain swelling may occur in response to a sharp blow. The collapse of some of the veins in the area may provide a few milliliters of needed space. In this way, the cerebral veins act as a buffer for ICV.

But the intracranial blood volume (IBV) can be reduced quite substantially — perhaps by 30 or 40 percent — by certain manipulations. It has been known for many years that *hyperventilation* will reduce ICP. We have seen previously that the pre-capillary arterioles, the capillaries, and probably the post-capillary venules — the so-called "capacitance vascular bed" of the brain — respond to lowering of the pCO_2 of the blood by vasoconstriction. Thus, intentional hyperventilation can induce a volume buffer for ICV.

Certain chemicals are capable of the same thing. Drugs such as the barbiturates, lidocaine, and alpha-thesin may cause an immediate and profound drop in ICP. It seems most likely that such agents cause intracranial vasoconstriction through a hypothalamic sympathetic reflex. Remember that a reduction in intracranial blood volume does not necessarily mean a fall in cerebral blood flow, nor a reduction in oxygen availability for the brain. Cerebral blood flow is linked to cerebral perfusion pressure by the autoregulation curve. However, it is fair to say that in areas of the brain where the autoregulation mechanism is not operative, attempted manipulations of the IBV may have no effect upon local blood volume.

There is some evidence that barbiturates may have a secondary protective effect on the brain, by reducing the neurone's requirements for oxygen. And thiopental, a very rapidly-acting barbituate, may, by virtue of the configuration of its sulphydryl group, act as a "sponge" to remove certain toxic products of oxygen metabolism, the oxygen-derived free radicals. Such free radicals may exist in toxic concentrations in intercellular spaces in some areas of swollen, damaged brain.

b. Cerebrospinal Fluid (CSF)

Another component of ICV that can be reduced readily is the CSF in the ventricles and the subarachnoid space. To some extent, this buffer system functions automatically. Every time you raise your ICP precipitously by coughing or sneezing or lifting something heavy — by suddenly increasing intrathoracic pressure and venous back-pressure into the head — you squirt a little extra CSF out of the ventricles or surface subarachnoid spaces into the spinal canal.

There is only one means for safely removing CSF from a patient with head injury, and that is by drainage of the ventricles. There is *no* indication for doing lumbar punctures on such patients, and the risks of doing so are substantial. The reason for this has to do with the partial compartmentalization of the intracranial space. Peruse Figure 3A once again. The intracranial space is not a single cavity. Therefore, pressure differentials can build up inside the head. When an abnormal volume is added to one of the intracranial compartments, the pressure in that compartment will exceed that in the others. Since brain tissue is incompressible in acute situations, and if all of the buffering mechanisms available have been exhausted, the brain itself must move —"shift" is the term usually used. Such shifts in brain tissue often result in "herniation" of the brain into another cranial compartment. Brain tissue may herniate beneath the falx, or through the incisural opening of the tentorium. Herniated brain tissue often loses its blood supply and becomes infarcted. At the incisural notch, herniating temporal lobe tissue may exert pressure upon the brain stem, inducing a hemiplegia, or upon the third cranial nerve, causing a dilated and fixed pupil. More aspects of cerebral herniations will be discussed in section 5 of this chapter.

In any event, sudden withdrawal or leakage of CSF from the lumbar subarachnoid space can cause serious differences in intracranial compartmental pressure relationships, and may lead to the dreaded brain herniations. Even CSF withdrawal from the ventricles may allow for cerebellar tissue to herniate upwards, although this event is not encountered commonly. In addition, an indwelling line in a ventricle makes it easy to monitor the ICP.

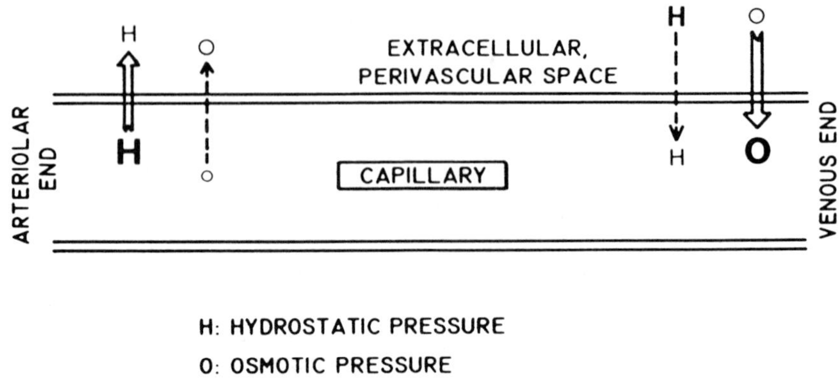

Figure 20. The principle of osmotherapy.

See text. When the osmotic pressure (0) at the arteriolar end of the capillary is increased greatly, by rapid infusion intravenously of a concentrated solution (such as 20% mannitol, 100 grams of mannitol dissolved in 500 ml water), the inward pull of the osmotic pressure overwhelms the normal balancing mechanisms of fluid out — fluid in along the capillary, sucking in a substantial volume of water.

c. Brain Water

The volume of water in the extravascular, extracellular space can be altered by a process known as *osmotherapy.* Fluids have an osmotic, or concentration, pressure that depends upon the number and types of certain molecules in the fluid.

If two fluids in a container are separated by a membrane that is permeable only to water, the fluid with the higher solute concentration will attract water to itself from the other compartment. There will be a tendency for the greater and the lesser concentrations to equilibrate at an intermediate value.

In the capillaries, a complex mechanism is seen. Figure 20 is a diagram of the situation. At the arteriolar end of the capillary, the principal force driving water and some solutes out of the vessel is hydrostatic pressure. The hydrostatic pressure dissipates quickly along the capillary, and at the venous end, the principal factor promoting water reabsorption into the capillary is the osmotic pressure.

If a solution with a very high concentration (such as a 20 percent solution of mannitol) is passed quickly through a capillary, the osmotic pressure difference between the intra- and the extravascular space is greatly enhanced. The effect will be to pull a large water volume from the extravascular spaces into the blood stream. Most of this water load will be excreted through the kidneys, producing a total body dehydrating effect.

All of this represents the physiological rationale for osmotherapy. The ideal osmotic agent would remain confined to the intravascular compartment, would be rapidly metabolized in the liver to non-toxic end products, and would dump all of its water load during its first circulation. Unfortunately, such an agent does not exist. There is always some leak of the agent into the extravascular compartment. If such a leak is great, as may occur in areas where the blood-brain barrier has broken down, quite rapidly the osmotic gradient between capillary and extravascular space may swing in favor of the latter. Then, "rebound" edema may occur. The prolonged use of osmotherapy, particularly in small children, may lead to severe problems in the management of water and electrolyte balance, to chronic dehydration, and occasionally to a hypovolemia-related mild hypoxemia. Nevertheless, osmotherapy is very useful in patients with traumatic cerebral edema and in those with expanding intracranial masses. Enough time may be gained by the temporary reduction in ICV that osmotherapy usually will produce for safe transport of the patient, for obtaining definitive diagnostic studies such as a CT scan, or for completion of proper operative procedures, while protecting brain function.

It will be obvious by now that the overriding concern in the manipulation of intracranial volume and intracranial pressure is the preservation of as much brain function as possible. Because of the closed-box features of the skull, during episodes of rapid increase in ICV, time is of the essence. When the brain is in jeopardy because of ICP or lack of metabolic substrate, time equals function. Cavalier or dithering attitudes toward the patient's status lead to catastrophe.

5. DELAYED DETERIORATION OF CONSCIOUSNESS

The archetypic lesion associated with delayed deterioration of consciousness is the extradural hematoma. Figures 21 and 22 are dramatic illustrations of what occurs during the evolution of such a blood clot, and Figure 23 is an actual post-mortem example.

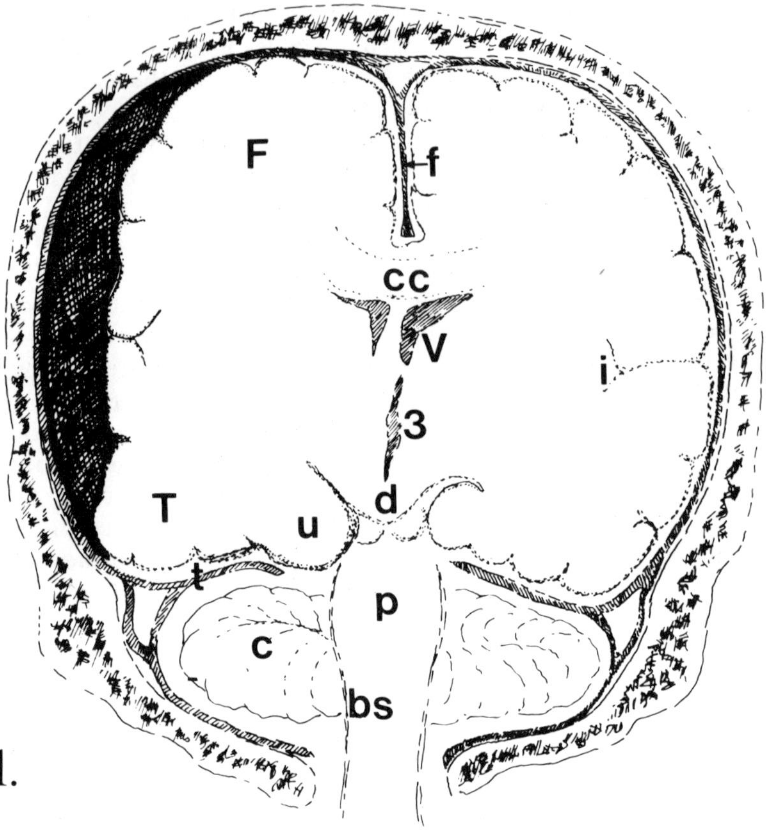

21.

Figures 21 and 22. The evolution of an extracerebral hematoma.

F — frontal lobe
T — temporal lobe
V — lateral ventricle
3 — third ventricle
f — falx
t — tentorium
i — insula
u — uncus of temporal lobe
p — pons
c — cerebellum
cc — corpus callosum
bs — lower brain stem
d — diencephalon (upper brain stem)
to — cerebellar tonsil

In this case, a subdural hematoma of arterial origin is enlarging on the surface of the right cerebral hemisphere. The effect is the same for an extradural clot.

In Figure 21, note that there is shift of the falx, some compression of the right lateral ventricle, early tilting of the corpus callosum, tilting of the third ventricle and diencephalon, and some displacement of the lower brain stem to the left. The uncus of the right temporal lobe has moved medially. It

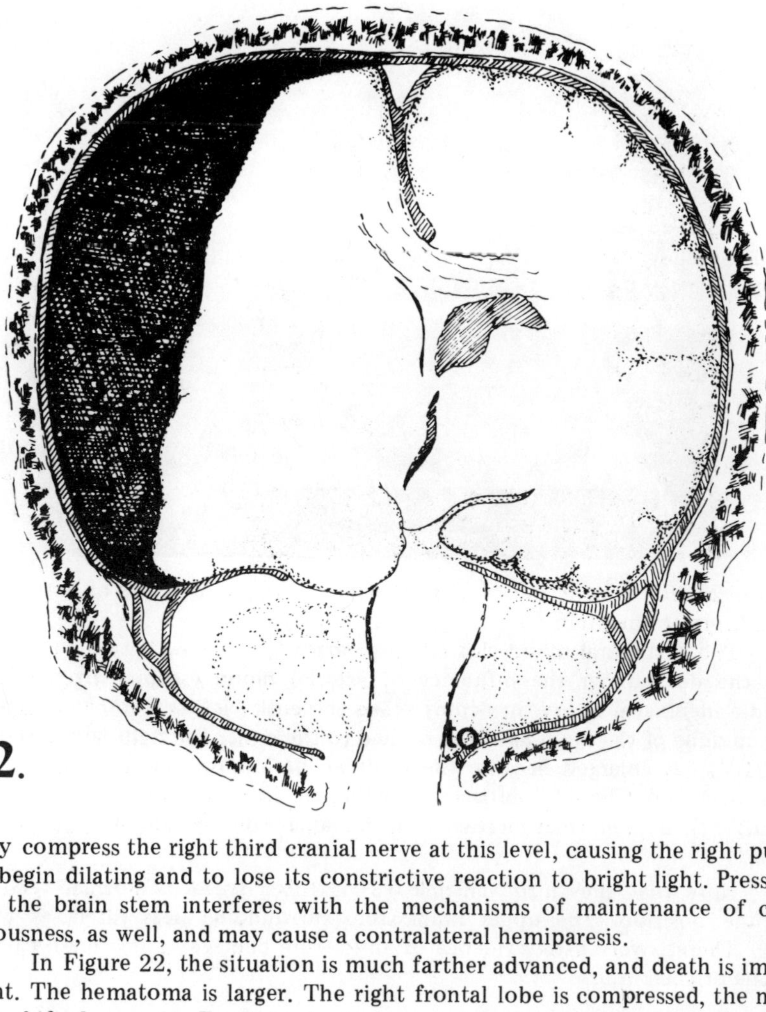

22.

may compress the right third cranial nerve at this level, causing the right pupil to begin dilating and to lose its constrictive reaction to bright light. Pressure on the brain stem interferes with the mechanisms of maintenance of consciousness, as well, and may cause a contralateral hemiparesis.

In Figure 22, the situation is much farther advanced, and death is imminent. The hematoma is larger. The right frontal lobe is compressed, the midline shifted severely. Frontal lobe tissue may have herniated beneath the falx. The right lateral ventricle is collapsed. Shift of the midline has occluded the left foramen of Monroe, and the left lateral ventricle is dilating.

Much more uncal herniation has occurred. The tentorial edge on the left is cutting into the midbrain. This will produce a hemiplegia on the right side of the body. By now, the patient will demonstrate stereotyped posturing on the left side.

Note that the contents of the left posterior fossa are compressed. This may lead to herniation of the cerebellar tonsil through the foramen magnum. Such an event usually compromises the control of breathing. Only immediate evacaution of the hematoma now carries any hope for the patient's survival.

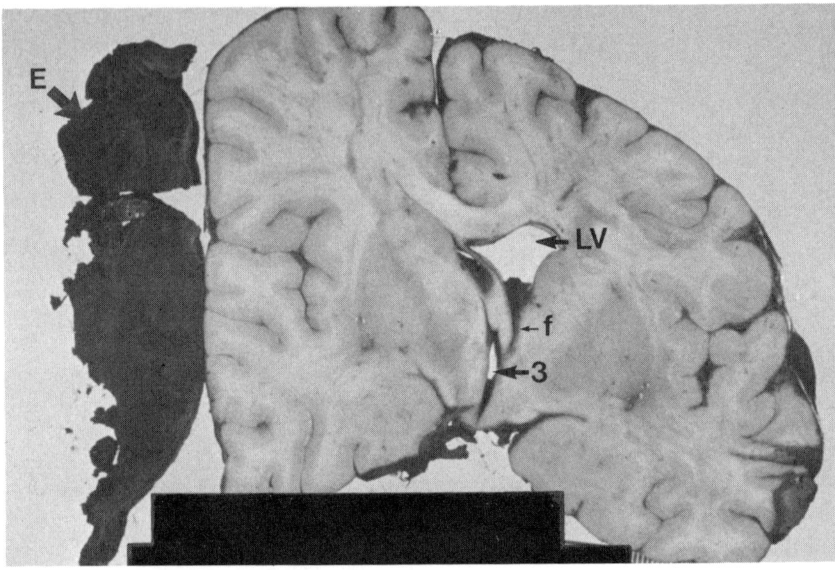

Figure 23. Reconstruction of post-mortem example of effect of extradural hematoma on the brain.

The extradural blood clot (E, large arrow), enlarging between the skull and the dura under the influence of arterial blood escaping from a torn middle meningeal artery, has compressed the entire left cerebral hemisphere. The midline of the brain has been pushed to the right. The right lateral ventricle (LV) has enlarged because the foramen of Monroe on the right (f) has been occluded. The left ventricle has collapsed in an attempt to compensate ("buffer") the abnormal increase in intracranial volume caused by the hematoma.

Note that the third ventricle (3) is tilted from its normal vertical, midline position. The upper brain stem surrounding it is tilted, as well.

There is very little evidence of any severe damage to this brain caused by the original injury.

In general, the sooner after the head injury the deterioration in the conscious state begins, and the more rapidly it progresses, the more critical is the situation for the patient.

When a hemorrhage such as is shown in Figure 25 occurs at or within seconds of the head impact, the patient is unconscious and remains so from the onset. But occasionally, the mass lesion may not begin to grow for many minutes, hours, even days. Of course, the damage to the blood vessel occurs at the moment of injury. An artery such as the middle meningeal (Figure 4A), may be torn, the bleeding may stop within seconds. Before the small blood clot that has sealed the artery has time to consolidate and harden, it is knocked off — perhaps by a fit of coughing, by vigorous head motion, or by sheer perversity. Often, the patient has wakened and may show no neurological deficit. Then he grows drowsier, he may develop a hemiplegia and a fixed pupil. If the situation is not corrected he will go on to stereotyped motor posturing, his breathing pattern may change and become inefficient, and he is in imminent danger of dying. Incisural herniation of brain tissue produces distortion of the brain stem, and traction upon and rupture of small perforating brain stem arteries may occur, producing a picture such as shown in Figure 24. The legends to Figures 21 and 22 are descriptive of this process, known to clinical neuroscientists as "rostro-caudal deterioration."

Blood clots such as those illustrated in Figures 25 and 26 usually reach maximum volumes within minutes of the injury. Seldom do the victims regain useful, independent function in such cases; even if they survive, the extent of original brain injury usually is very great. Such clots often occur in the absence of skull fractures.

The potential tragedy of the extradural hematoma is that the patient is completely salvageable, usually. The bleeding arises outside of the dura and the brain may have sustained little or no tissue damage at the moment of impact. Critical delay in the recognition of what is happening leads to the process shown in Figures 21, 22, and 24. In 90 percent or more of such patients, a skull fracture is found on skull x-ray. But in infancy, fully one third of all extradural hematomas occur in the absence of skull fracturing. You will appreciate now that the presence of absence of a skull fracture is a poor hook upon which to hang an estimation of the potential seriousness of a head injury.

There are other causes of delayed deterioration of consciousness. The development of *vasogenic cerebral edema* may create a mass effect locally or more diffusely. Usually such edema arises because of damage to blood vessels in the injured brain, but certain therapeutic measures may encourage its growth.

You will recall our discussion of cerebral perfusion pressure (CPP) in Section 2 of this chapter. We emphasized the need for maintaining a critical CPP to the brain if cerebral infarction is to be avoided. Work recently completed in our Brain Research Laboratory (London, Ont.) strongly suggests that *too high* CPP promotes the formation of more vasogenic edema in injured areas.

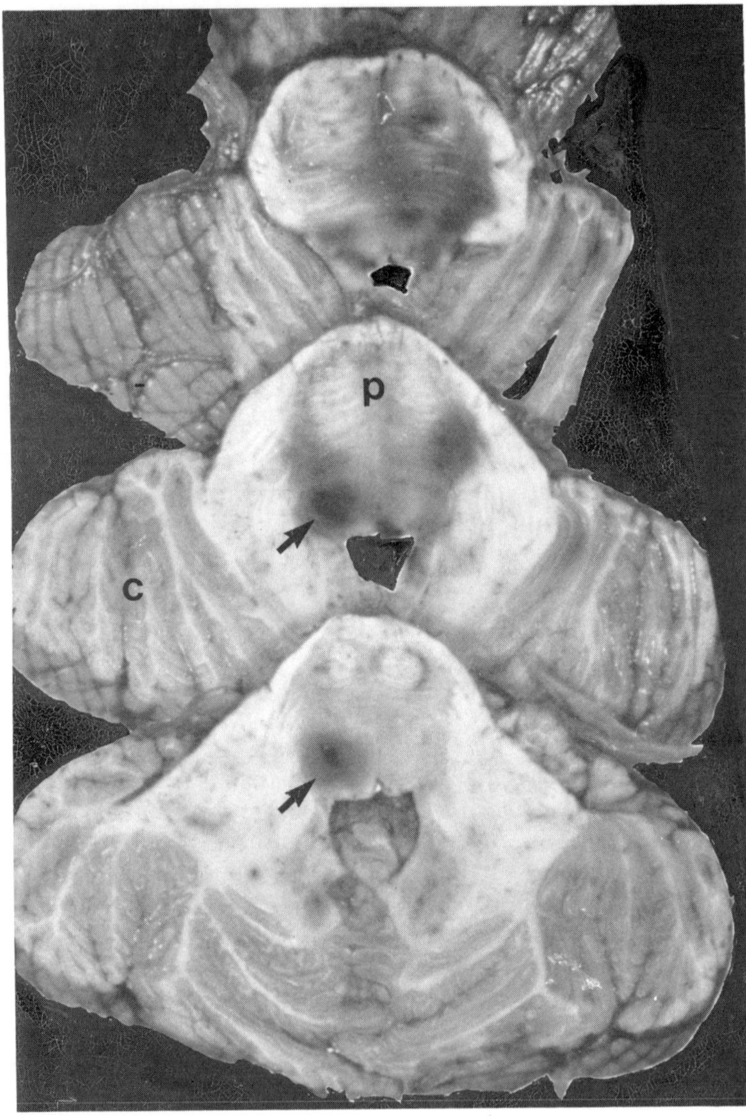

Figure 24. Horizontal sections through the brain stem, level of pons.

Arrows indicate hemorrhages into the pons (p). In this example, the blood clots are in the part of the pons that contains elements of the ascending reticular activating system (aras). The patient was in coma from the moment of impact, and never woke up. The cerebellum (c) is relatively undamaged.

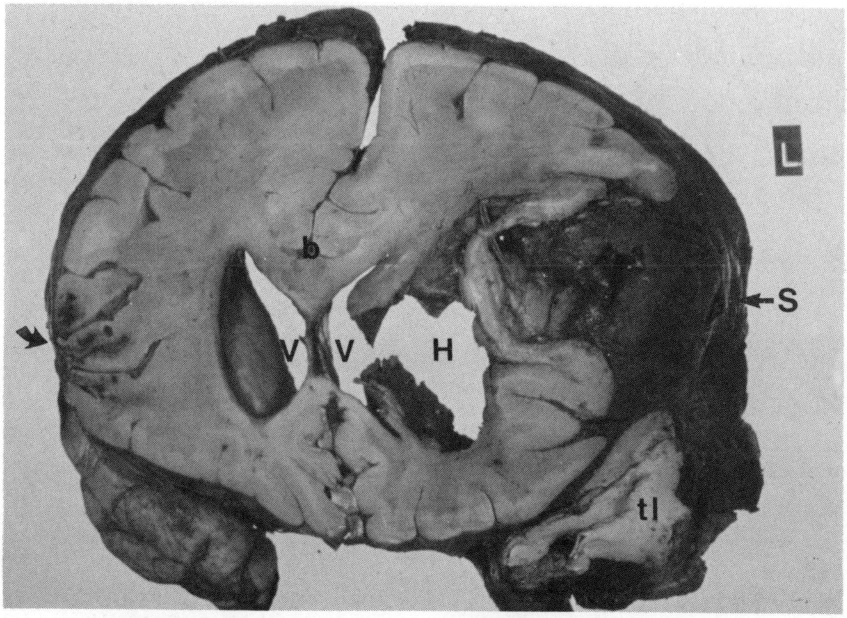

Figure 25. Post-mortem brain section, trauma.

In this patient, the impact occurred on the left side of the head. S marks an acute subdural hematoma. The sliver is in a brain laceration through which the subdural clot was in continuity with an intracerebral clot (H). The intracerebral clot had ruptured into the left lateral ventricle (V), and both ventricles were filled with and dilated by blood. The clot has fallen out of V and H during preparation.

Bruising of the cerebral cortex remote from the site of impact is seen in the right frontal cortex (curved arrow), in the tip of the left temporal lobe (tl), and in the corpus callosum, just below b. Note how much shift of the midline has occurred.

It was impossible to be certain which blood clot (H or S) was the primary event. For a clot to rip brain apart as shown here, the bleeding must be arterial in origin.

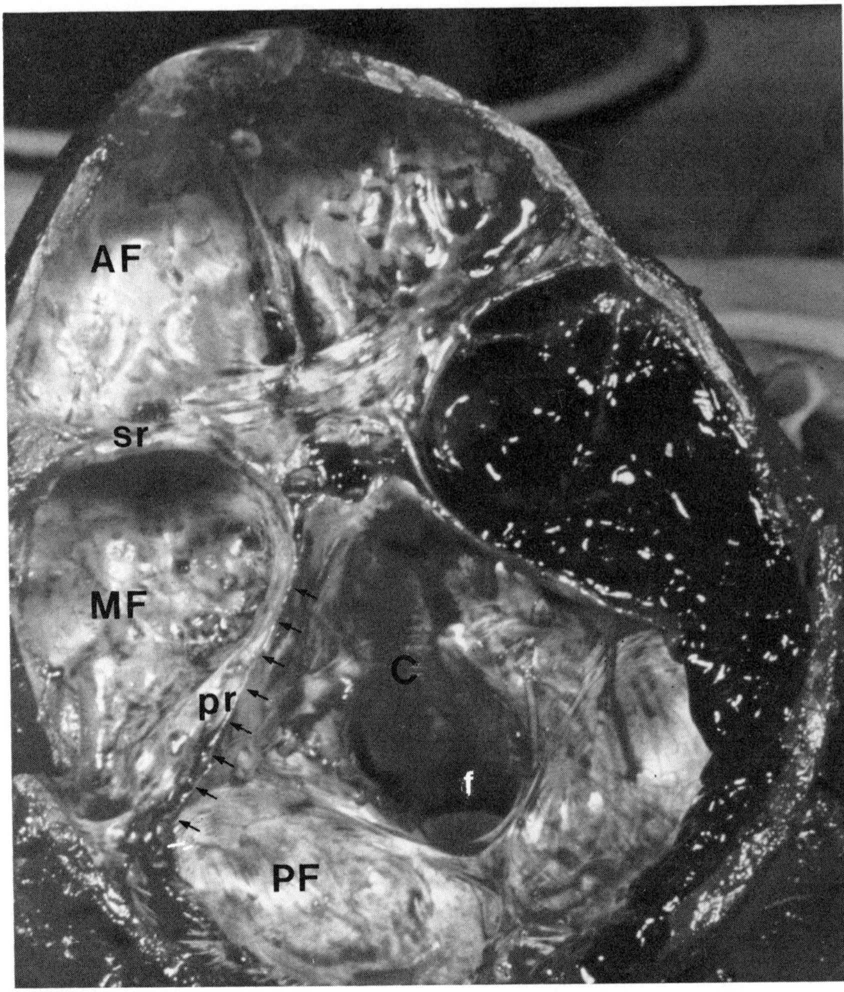

Figure 26. Post-mortem view of base of skull, showing an acute subdural hematoma.

Note the roughness of the floor of the anterior fossa (AF), the sickle-like shape and sharpness of the sphenoid ridge (sr), and the sloping, rough faces of the petrous ridge (pr). The line of arrows indicates the point of attachment of the tentorium, here removed, that supports the occipital lobes and separates the supratentorial space — anterior (AF) and middle (MF) fossae — from the posterior fossa (PF).

The right middle fossa is filled with fresh blood clot. Note the fresh blood lying on the clivus (C), the anterior wall of the posterior fossa. The foramen magnum (f) is the place where brain stem becomes spinal cord.

Manipulation of the intracranial volume buffer system may ameliorate the mass effects of cerebral edema, but if the blood vessels in the injured area have lost autoregulation and/or the blood brain barrier, the surgeon really is treating only the normal brain. There is no incontrovertible evidence in the literature that supports the administration of steroids for the reduction of traumatic cerebral edema. One hopes to stop the spread of edema and to gain sufficient time for the situation to correct itself. The use of more heroic measures such as profound hypothermia and barbiturate coma have advocates, but there is no satisfactory evidence that they consistently alter outcome.

Fat and *bone-marrow emboli* may interfere with the cerebral microcirculation following major orthopedic injury. Very often there are severe pulmonary effects as well, further interfering with proper oxygen transport to neurones. Overwhelming fat embolism usually induces an intractible and fatal cerebral edema. Petechial hemorrhages occur in the brain, the retinae, and sclera, the kidneys, the skin. Heparin infusion and extremely vigorous therapy for cerebral edema may be successful in averting tragedy.

In Chapter 3 we saw how the cerebrospinal fluid (CSF) is produced at a steady rate of 0.35 ml per minute, and that its production ceases only when ICP exceeds CPP. When blood is spilled into the subarachnoid space, obstruction of the CSF outflow pathways may occur. The ventricles may begin to dilate. This condition is called *post-traumatic hydrocephalus*, and if it occurs rapidly enough, it adds materially to any mass effect within the head. Further, distortion of the ventricular system itself may cause ventricular enlargement in varying combinations (Figures 21, 22 and 25). Figure 23 graphically illustrates the so-called "double mass" effect of a blood clot on one side, and an obstructed ventricle on the other. The dilating ventricle compounds the problem by acting as a second mass lesion. Post-traumatic hydrocephalus is an important cause of secondary deterioration. Drainage of the offending ventricle(s) will obviate at least *that* part of the situation. When extensive scarring occurs in the subarachnoid spaces because of traumatic subarachnoid hemorrhage, the ensuing hydrocephalus may be permanent. An implanted system of tubes and valves, a CSF shunt, then may be required for ongoing control of the hydrocephalus.

Occasionally, the subarachnoid space may become infected following head injury. Such *infection* is likely to occur when a basal skull fracture produces a communication between an air-filled sinus such as the frontal sinus, and the subarachnoid space. An acute bacterial meningitis may ensue. Such an infection may cause permanent CSF obstruction as well, with hydrocephalus as its consequence.

Trauma to the central nervous system (CNS) even when quite mild, on rare occasions will induce an abnormal water-balance state by mechanisms unknown, or by severance of the stalk of the pituitary gland. The syndromes may be associated with severe hypo- or hypernatremia, and either situation may interfere with brain function. Seizures may develop, as well.

Finally, injury to other parts of the body may contribute to or cause a late deterioration in brain function. Hypovolemic shock and lung injury with hypoxemia are of major importance. Mild cerebral edema will be aggravated by cerebral hypoxemia or ischemia.

Occasional individuals react to stress by becoming hyperglycemic, even to blood sugar levels that may cause coma. Some other phenomena rarely seen include severe hypophosphatemia that may simulate brain death, and severe stress diuresis that may produce a hyperosmolar state with altered consciousness and seizures.

6. LATE DETERIORATION IN NEUROLOGICAL FUNCTION

Sometimes, changes in CNS function that are definitely related to brain trauma do not appear for days, weeks, or even months. This classical example of this situation is the *chronic subdural hematoma.* This space-taking lesion usually occurs on one side only, high on the brain convexity. The most likely mechanism is a small amount of venous bleeding onto the brain surface at the time of injury, a volume of blood that clots. As the clotted blood begins to break up, a fluid-solid mixture is formed. Irritation of the undersurfaces of the dura by blood leads to fibroblast proliferation and formation of a vascular membrane. After three weeks or so, membranes will line both the outer and the inner aspects of the lesion.

Why the chronic subdural hematoma expands in some patients is uncertain. Quite often, a small volume of fresh subdural blood will be absorbed over a few days or weeks. In other cases, the lesion begins to produce symptoms (mild hemiparesis, headache, personality change, seizures) after days, weeks, or months. Earlier thoughts that the hematoma exerts an osmotic attractive force have not survived critical investigations. It is likely that the membrane bleeds a little at intervals, adding to the cumulative volume and to the pressure upon the brain surface. Simple drainage of the hematoma is curative in most cases.

Occasionally, the subdural collection is blood-stained CSF under pressure. Here, the mechanism probably is a tear in the arachnoid and a ball-valve situation where brain pulsation pushes CSF into the subdural space, at the same time preventing its egress. Not infrequently, such *subdural effusions* become symptomatic within days of injury.

Because it may take weeks or months for the process of scar formation in the subarachnoid space following traumatic subarachnoid hemorrhage or meningitis to become severe enough to seriously compromise CSF flow, post-traumatic hydrocephalus must be considered when CNS function begins to deteriorate some time following the injury.

We must make a distinction between delayed deterioration in CNS function and delayed recognition that CNS function had been compromised much earlier. It is obvious that most tests of cortical function cannot be made until the patient is awake and cooperative. Some residual, perhaps permanent, signs of CNS damage may then become apparent. An example here might be a visual field defect, say, to the right. In a patient who has survived very high intracranial pressure waves or a herniation of the left temporal lobe that temporarily occluded the major blood supply to the visual occipital cortex on the left, such a finding might be expected.

7. BRAIN DEATH

Yogi Berra once commented that "it ain't over until the fat lady sings." For the human organism, it's all over once the cerebral hemispheres have been deprived of blood supply for long enough to cause irreversible and irrecoverable damage to the cortex, the repository of all that makes us human.

The identification of brain death still is principally a clinical event. Most jurisdictions insist upon absence of brain stem reflexes and of peripheral response to stimulation — other than purely spinal reflexes — before such a statement can be made if life-support is to be suspended. A totally flat EEG, recorded over at least 30 minutes, may be required as well.

Cerebral contrast angiography or radionuclide dynamic brain scanning may show lack of cerebral hemisphere blood perfusion even in the presence of retention of some brain stem reflexes. Such a situation is never compatible with any sort of functional recovery, and does in fact signify brain death. This issue is more than academic because of the desperate need for organ donors. Early recognition of brain death will make more undamaged organs available for transplantation.

In this chapter, we have explored at some length certain mechanisms and pathophysiologic features of head injury. Next, we shall discuss the clinical spectrum of head trauma in children.

SOURCES AND READINGS

Apfelbaum RI, Guthkelch AN, Shulman K: Experimental production of subdural hematomas. *J Neurosurg 40:* 336–346, 1974.

Bruce DA: *The Pathophysiology of Increased Intracranial Pressure.* Current Concepts, Upjohn, 1978.

Durward QJ, Delmaestro RF, Amacher AL, Ferrar JK: The influence of systemic arterial pressure and intracranial pressure on the development of cerebral vasogenic edema. *J Neurosurg 59:* 803–809, 1983.

Gurdjian ES: Recent advances in the study of the mechanism of impact injury of the head - a summary. *Clin Neurosurg 19:* 1–42, 1972.

Strich SJ: Cerebral Trauma. In *Greenfield's Neuropathology.* 3rd Ed., Edward Arnold, London, 1976. Chapter 9.

Strich SJ: Shearing of nerve fibres as a cause of brain damage due to head injury. A pathological study of twenty cases. *Lancet 2:* 443–448, 1961.

Takagi H, Tamaki Y, Morii S, Ohwada T: Rapid enlargement of ventricles within seven hours after head injury. *Surg Neurol 16:* 103–105, 1981.

Weir B: The osmolality of subdural hematoma fluid. *J Neurosurg 34:* 528–533, 1971.

Zimmerman RA, Bilaniuk LT, Bruce D, Dolinskas C, Obrist W, Kuhl D: Computed tomography of pediatric head trauma: acute general cerebral swelling. *Radiology 126:* 403–408, 1978.

CHAPTER 5

The Clinical Spectrum

1. BIRTH INJURY

The journey down the birth canal may be the most hazardous that a child will ever make. Admittedly, the recent advances in obstetrical techniques and the earlier resort to Cesarean section in obstructed labors have reduced greatly the incidence of serious CNS injuries to the neonate. Still, certain injuries crop up with sufficient frequency to merit our attention. Some of these are likely to require ongoing physiotherapy, remedial surgery, or corrective appliances. It is easier to explore this topic according to the obstetrical presentation of the child and the delivery technique employed.

a. Vertex (Head) Presentations, Forceps Deliveries

The misapplication of obstetrical forceps occurs occasionally. Usually, a *linear skull fracture* often accompanied by a hematoma beneath the scalp or the periosteum of the cranial bone (usually the parietal) results. Most of these are of little consequence, although a very large scalp hematoma may produce a significant drop in the baby's hemoglobin concentration. Analagous to skull fracture is a "sprung" suture line; the cause is the same.

Sometimes the skull fracture is *depressed.* Classically, this fracture resembles a pushed-in ping-pong ball, hence the name "ping-pong fracture." These are easily corrected.

Not all skull fractures during labor are the fault of forceps. Some years ago, Eban Alexander and the group at Winston–Salem showed that the pounding of the infant head on the sacral promontory during hard labor could cause linear or depressed fractures.

More serious are basal skull fractures involving the petrous ridges, the auditory canals, often the auditory and facial nerves.

Severe disruption of a petrous ridge may cause a CSF leak, a permanent loss of hearing, and a permanent facial palsy on the affected side. Such injuries may occur when all due care is taken; most frequently they happen when less experienced people attempt to turn a baby from a transverse or occiput posterior lie to the normal occiput anterior presentation, misapplying the forceps in the process.

Facial nerve injuries often occur in the absence of a skull fracture. Here, the tip of the forceps blade digs into the baby's cheek just in front of and below the ear. All too often the damage is permanent.

The commonly seen bi-parietal posterior swellings are of no concern. They occur in the absence of forceps application, and probably are a normal concommitant of head-moulding during delivery.

b. Vertex Presentations, Impacted Shoulders

Few things can spur infrequent or inexperienced operators to panic as quickly as the large infant whose shoulders has become impacted behind the symphysis pubis, particularly when the fetal heart rate begins to slow. Pulling down the head, with rotation, in order to relieve this *shoulder dystocia*, is very likely to stretch elements of the *brachial plexus*, that network of sensory and motor nerve fibres passing to and from the cervical spinal cord and the arm. If the nerve fibres are stretched to the point that they rupture, a permanent palsy of the arm will ensue. The exact pattern of paralysis is variable, but two principal types are seen. The situation depicted above usually causes damage to the upper part of the brachial plexus, resulting in paralysis of the muscles of the shoulder and arm. The child has a nearly normal hand, but she cannot get it to her mouth or head. Loss of neurotropic influences upon young muscles results in atrophy and arm shortening. Without expert physiotherapy, shoulder and elbow joints will develop contractures with severe loss of mobility and chronic pain. The eponym attached to this entity is "Erb's paralysis." It is a very serious disability.

If the operator attempts to disengage the impacted shoulder by inserting a finger under the arm into the axilla and spinning the child, the damage from a too-deeply inserted finger may be to the lower part of the brachial plexus. Here, the brunt of the paralysis falls upon the hand and wrist muscles. This is "Klumpke's paralysis." Even if it sounds more devastating than the Erb's type, it is not. Almost always, the hand retains useful — even normal — sensation. The upper arm is normal or nearly so, so the extremity remains very useful and nearly totally mobile. Again, proper physiotherapy enhances the final result. I see three or four brachial plexus injuries per year. Since there is nothing that I, a surgeon, can do to repair torn proximal nerve fibres, I hustle the little people directly — the same day — to the pediatric physiotherapists. What they can accomplish under such circumstances with their programs of home and outpatient therapy, concentrating upon joint mobility and strengthening of intactly innervated muscles, has never ceased to amaze me. These children should not end up as cripples, disabled though they may be.

The most feared complication of traction upon a head in the case of shoulder dystocia is best described with the next entity.

c. Breech Deliveries

Desperate though the consequences of improperly managed vertex presentations may be, they pale in the face of the horrors that may occur when a baby emerges breech. Here, the legs and rump are delivered first. Sometimes the umbilical cord slips out, as well. Any compression of the umbilical cord will shut off oxygen supply to the infant. The infant heart will slow dramatically. If panic is commonly the spectre with shoulder impaction, it is the rule with such a breech delivery. At this point there is no alternative: the infant must be delivered quickly. The impulse is to start pulling.

As is the rule in such circumstances, the baby is usually pelvis-down relative to the mother. Traction upon the baby's torso tends to cause extension of the head behind the pubis, increasing the obstruction and the panic on the part of the operator. Unfortunately, the intra-spinous ligaments, the intervertebral discs and the spinal cord of the newborn are not meant to withstand very much longitudinal stretching force. The cervical spinal cord may be pulled entirely apart. If this occurs above the C4 or C5 segments, the baby will not breathe and usually will die promptly. If it happens below that level, the baby will be quadriplegic — one of the items on the differential diagnosis list for the "floppy infant." I have seen one instance in which four centimeters of cervical spinal cord were totally replaced by fibrous tissue. There are cases on record in which the child's head has been physically separated from the torso.

Breech delivery is not something to be undertaken lightly.

d. Babies With Very Large Heads

At the present, there is little excuse for attempting to deliver babies with congenital, intra-uterine hydrocephalus vaginally. Except in instances where the mother has eschewed prenatal care, the obstetrician should be aware of perinatal hydrocephalus. Polyhydramnios, unusual lies, failure of the first stage of labor, should prompt ultrasonic exploration of the uterus and its contents.

In times gone by, it was not unusual for an obstetrician to find himself suddenly faced with a grossly distended intra-uterine head. Often, his only recourse was to insert a trocar into the anterior fontanelle, decompress the head by drainage, and deliver the child. Seldom did the infant live long.

Recently, I reported upon four infants known to have intrauterine hydrocephalus between 32 and 40 weeks of fetal life (Child's Brain). Our approach in those infants was (1) ensure lung maturity by amniocentesis, (2) delivery by Cesarean section electively, (3) CSF shunt very early in life (1-12 days). With a minimum follow-up now of 2.5 years, three of the four are totally normal.

Others have begun to insert CSF shunts in utero in such babies, under ultrasonic and radiographic control, draining CSF into the amniotic fluid. My experience has been that babies hydrocephalic in utero should be given a chance. The practice of inserting a trocar into the heads of such infants during delivery should now be a regrettable — though necessary — thing of the past.

2. CONCUSSIVE INJURIES

a. The Common Triad

Almost every child who sustains a significant blow to the head, whether unconscious or not, will exhibit what I call the "common triad." Shortly after the incident, he will become *drowsy*, want to lie down and sleep. If disturbed, he will be *irritable* and unreasonable. He will complain of *nausea*, and will usually vomit, not once or twice, but repeatedly. After a severe head injury, of course, he will remain unconscious, with the manifestations of head injury at any age. For our purposes now, we consider only the so-called "trivial" head injury.

It is usually the drowsiness and nausea that prompt parents to seek assistance. Sometimes the vomiting is pernicious enough to require intravenous replacement. By the next morning, both the drowsiness and nausea usually have disappeared. Easy fatiguability and shortness of temper may persist for several days, even weeks. Older children may complain that bright light and loud sounds bother them, and that they have trouble concentrating. Post-traumatic headaches are uncommon in children, but are encountered with increasing frequency through the adolescent years. These latter symptoms comprise the post-traumatic syndrome, and will be discussed in more detail later.

b. Skull Fractures

The younger the child, the thinner are the skull bones, and the more likely are they to fracture with any given force. There is usually a scalp hematoma associated. Fractures commonly occur with childhood head injury, and the knowledge that their child has a skull fracture is very worrisome to many parents. Most of them are of no consequence, but some merit close observation or surgical correction.

1) Fractures crossing vascular channels. The middle meningeal artery and its two major branches, and the large venous sinuses, may be lacerated by linear or depressed fractures. Either may produce extradural, and the latter may be the origin of subdural, bleeding. Figure 27 is an example of a dangerous fracture overlying venous sinuses.

2) Depressed fractures. A fracture is said to be depressed if one edge, or one part of a comminuted lesion, is pushed in more than the width of the skull. Sometimes the dura and even the cortex directly beneath is lacerated. In general, depressed fractures should be repaired. Most certainly they should if they overlie the primary motor, sensory, or speech areas of the cortex.

3) Open fractures, whether depressed or not, must be surgically debrided and the scalp closed. They represent avenues for bacteria into the head. If definitive treatment of the fracture must be delayed for any reason, it is quite proper to close the laceration loosely, controlling all bleeding points. Infants and children

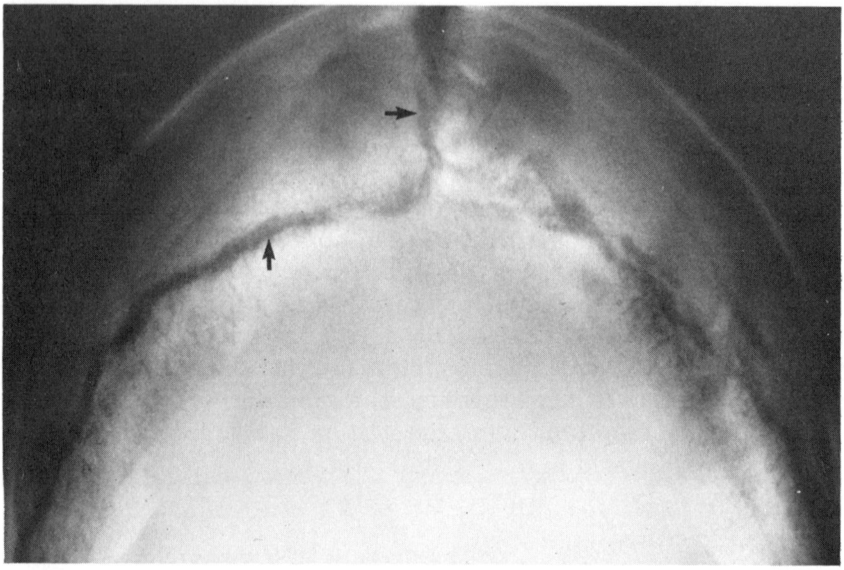

Figure 27. Skull fractures overlying venous sinuses.

This close-up radiograph of the posterior skull shows a dangerous fracture directly overlying the sagittal sinus (horizontal arrow) and the transverse sinus (vertical arrow). If the dural wall of the sinus is torn at the time of impact, a venous extradural clot may form, or a large hematoma beneath the scalp. In a young child, blood loss from such an injury may be sufficient to cause hemodynamic shock.

can lose a great deal of blood from oozing lacerations of the scalp, even to the point of hypovolemic shock.

4) Basal skull fractures into air-filled sinuses, with cerebrospinal fluid leak, are worrisome. The potential for CSF infection is present. Air may enter the head through frontal or ethomoidal sinus fractures. Loss of substantial volumes of CSF through the nose or ear may induce a low-pressure state intracranially, with severe headache.

It is seldom necessary to surgically close a CSF leak from the ear; almost all will dry up on their own. However, nasal leaks that persist for more than a few days should be explored and sealed.

The prophylactic use of antibiotics with CSF leaks following trauma is a debatable point. Critical evidence mitigates against their use, for the normal flora of the sinus or middle ear will be disrupted and an intracranial infection, if it occurs, will be due to a resistant organism that may be very virulent.

Loss of smell may occur with frontal basal fractures. In the case of fractures involving the ear, the bony ossicles of the middle ear may be dislocated causing a conductive and correctable deafness, but damage to the inner ear produces a permanent nerve deafness. CSF filling the middle ear always causes a temporary conductive deafness. It is my practice to have all children with temporal bone petrous fractures examined by an ear specialist.

Basal fractures rarely injure other cranial nerves, such as the sixth (abduction of the eye) or seventh (facial nerve). When the fracture involves the posterior orbit, damage may occur to the optic nerve and to the nerves of ocular motility.

5) Widened (diastatic) fractures are always dangerous. Their presence signifies raised intracranial pressure. When such a fracture is seen in association with a boggy scalp mass and an appropriate neurological deficit, it must be assumed that there is a brain laceration until proven otherwise.

If a diastatic skull fracture exists with a dural laceration below, an intact arachnoid membrane may bulge out into the fracture. Then, under the persistent pulsatile ebb and flow of the CSF into the arachnoid hernia, the fracture may start to grow. An extreme example of such a *growing fracture* is presented in Figure 28. At operation, a huge surface arachnoid cyst was resected, an artificial dura was inserted, and the bone defect had to be closed with an acrylic/wire-mesh cranioplasty.

6) Indriven bone fragments caused by perforating injuries should be removed, as the risk of contamination of the bone chips is quite high (30-50%). It may take a very long time for trouble to arise; brain abscess formation about a retained bone chip may be delayed for months, even years, from the original injury.

This litany of troubles associated with skull fractures may seem to give the lie to the statement earlier that most such are of no consequence. In a personal series of 862 head-injured children deemed not to be severely hurt but admitted to hospital, 338 had skull fractures (39.2%). Of those 338, 83 were complicated by being depressed or open, requiring surgical attention (24.5%). In other words, three-quarters of the skull fractures had no bearing upon the outcome for the child. At the same time, only 4 of the 524 patients without fractures in this group went on to develop intracranial mass lesions requiring operation (0.76%).

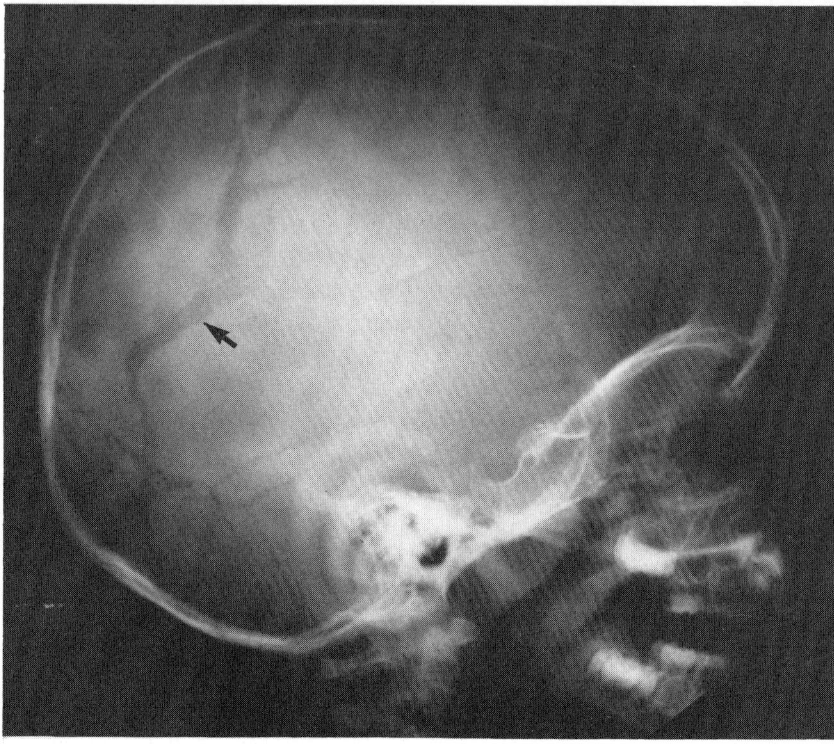

Figure 28A. Diastatic skull fracture.

This infant fell against a table-top edge. He had a boggy scalp mass and a hemiparesis. At the first operation, there was a laceration of dura and brain. The dural repair was inadequate.

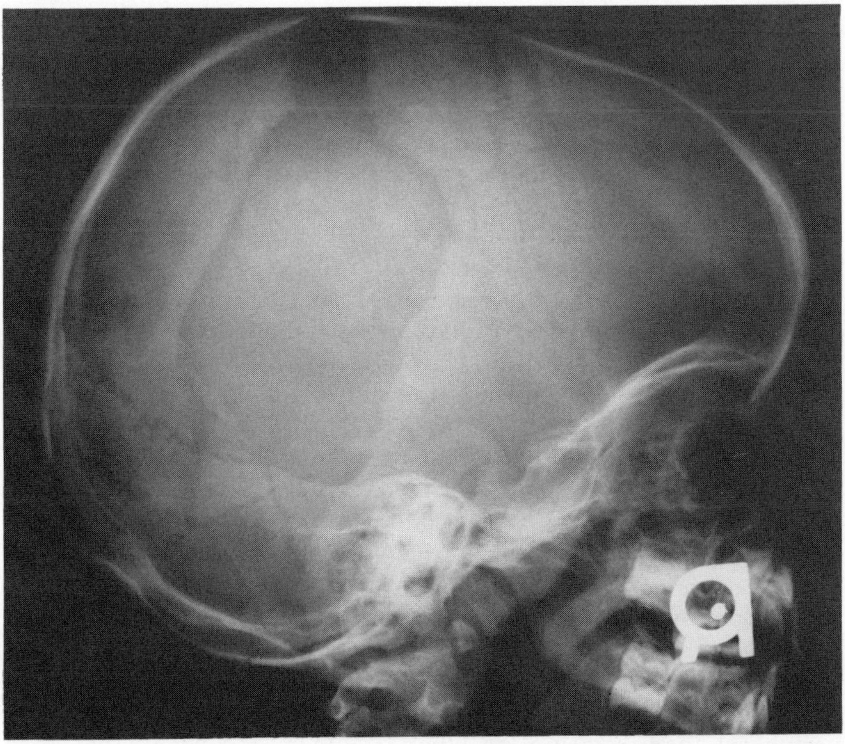

Figure 28B. Growing skull fracture.

Over a period of months, the boy developed a large, tense mass beneath the scalp. This x-ray shows that the original fracture has grown enormously. Herniation of the subarachnoid space into a fracture line allows the incessant pulsations of the brain transmitted by the CSF to erode the bone edges.

c. Seizures and Epilepsy

Children quite frequently have a seizure immediately or shortly after a head injury. My experience suggests that about 7% of children and adolescents do. This seizure rate, interestingly, is the same as that reported from the Hospital for Sick Children in Toronto in 1964, from a series of over 4,000 head-injured children. The incidence declines with age. Very seldom, in the absence of brain laceration or extensive contusion, does the occurrence have any significance for the future.

In 40% of the seizure cases, the fit occurs immediately. Only 9 or 10% of children who do have a post-traumatic seizure will do so after the third day. It is of interest that the longer the post-traumatic seizure is delayed, the more likely it is to lead to ongoing trouble.

Why younger children seem to be more susceptible to post-traumatic seizures is unknown. A common suggestion is that it reflects incomplete cerebral myelin insulation of nerve fibres, or, as yet incomplete synaptic contact with inhibitory neurones, in particular.

Experimental head injury models indicate that at the moment of significant head impact, a massive electrical discharge occurs. Perhaps, in the individual with a lower threshold for dampening the seizure discharge, this occurrence predisposes to a peripheral manifestation of what occurs in the brain, that is, a seizure that is clinically manifest.

In any case, the post-traumatic seizure often frightens the stuffing out of anyone who sees it. The principal point to make is: do not allow the patient to become hypoxic. The vast majority of such seizures are short-lived. Very seldom do they recur, and very seldom do they compromise the clinical status of the patient. Nor do such seizures imply that the child will become epileptic. It is extremely important to convey these realities to the parents.

Seizures, particularly focal ones, that have their onset many hours of days following the injury, may be the harbingers of the delayed onset of an intracranial mass lesion. This is especially so if the seizures are recurrent. Such a situation should prompt initial or repeat investigation, such as a CT scan.

There is probably a greater risk of the child having a seizure if she has sustained a localized cortical bruise, particularly over motor areas. Certainly, in a child with a depressed skull fracture over the cortical motor strip who has had a focal seizure, I regularly open the dura to inspect the brain surface. Not infrequently a surprise is revealed, such as a small surface clot, a surface laceration, an obvious contusion, even a subcortical intracerebral hematoma. In such instances it is wise to place the child on anticonvulsant medication for a period of three to six weeks.

I do not treat the usual post-traumatic seizure unless it is prolonged. There is debate on this point, but I have had no reason to change my approach. Most people would favor diazepam, 0.1 mgm per kilogram, as the most effective drug in such circumstances. Diazepam will, on occasion, induce a short apneic spell in a child upon intravenous bolus injection, especially in infants or in children on barbiturates. The simple appreciation of this fact should be sufficient to prevent panic if it occurs.

There is reason to believe that neurones discharging at abnormally high rates for long periods may burn themselves out, possibly on the basis of nutritional substrate failure and inability to produce synaptic chemical precursors. If the seizure interferes with proper pulmonary gas exchange, it is especially dangerous. Consequently, prolonged seizures and those that induce inefficient breathing patterns must be controlled quickly. A traumatized brain cannot tolerate the additional insult of hypoxia.

d. To Admit or Not

Any sort of analysis of pediatric head injuries based solely upon cost-benefit ratios would conclude that the overwhelming majority of children that have been or are now admitted to hospital following head injury need not have been or should not be admitted. My own experience confirms such a view. However, as a very wise man once remarked, medical statistics are nothing more than numbers of people with the tears removed. We are not dealing with cattle; we are dealing with human lives and with human concern.

It has been the practice on my service to send home as many children as possible following head injury. A degree of fine-tuning and sensibility is required here. If the child does not have a skull fracture — for all such are admitted for at least 24 hours — and if the parents feel comfortable with having the child home, getting up every hour during the night to check respiration and breathing pattern and ease of arousal, then home he goes. Fully one quarter as many children as the 862 mentioned previously have been sent home from the emergency room, on this basis. Only one has come to any grief, and that so slowly that the parents, properly alerted, returned him in ample time to forestall any sort of late consequence. It must be emphasized here that we are speaking only of those children whose initial examination by an experienced individual suggests that they will run no appreciable risk of disaster if they return home. Of the 524 children without skull fracture admitted to hospital, children whose examination in the emergency room suggested that they would come to no grief, only 4 went on to develop late mass lesions such as subdural hematoma or extradural hamatoma (0.76%). In every one of those cases the pathology developed slowly (4 to 7 days) and never became life-threatening prior to recognition.

Of the patients admitted with skull fractures, patients initially felt to have an insignificant head injury, 6 of 338 went on to die of intracranial catastrophes. This is an incidence of 1.8%. Three of these had been admitted to peripheral hospitals, deteriorated suddenly with extracerebral clots, and arrived at our unit in desperate condition. However, three children had been admitted directly to our unit, were improving for a time, then deteriorated very rapidly with overwhelming cerebral edema.

Therefore, one might conclude that the risk of serious trouble in children with so-called minor head injuries is very small — in my own series 10 of 862 or 1.2%, actually less than 1% if those children sent home from the emergency room are included.

The controversy pro and con regarding admission of such children to hospital for 24 or 48 hours observation will continue. The situation is much different for badly injured children, whether recognized initially or not. We shall explore that group in section 3 of this chapter.

e. Diagnostic Measures

Skull X-rays: Much has been made, usually by individuals who do not have to care for or worry about head-injured children, of the volume of apparently unnecessary skull radiographs that are obtained following apparently trivial concussions. Comments about "defensive medicine," "knee-jerk reactions" and so on, abound. The threat of malpractice suit as a motivating factor on the part of the physician is always mentioned.

To some extent, such attitudes have validity. In my own personal experience, the acquisition of skull films has been of any importance only in some 7 or 8% of cases.

However, these figures must be turned around. If even as few as 25% of skull fractures require surgical attention — and many of these are apparent because of an overlying laceration — even if that number is only 10%, the physician caring for the child should have the privilege of being able to estimate the odds. If one presents the facts to parents in these terms, the vast majority are in agreement with obtaining the films. The radiation exposure is negligible. It is my experience that children with skull fractures should be observed very closely for 24 to 48 hours. If the child seems safe, and there is no skull fracture, observation at home can be recommended with much greater confidence. Even an experienced pediatric neurosurgeon makes mistakes, but if the child has no skull fracture and the parents are responsible, the risk to a child who shows nothing more than the common triad head injury are miniscule if home observation is chosen.

CT Scan: To a variable extent, CT scanning is used as a substitute for common sense. Depending upon the machine, the radiation exposure may *not* be negligible. Certainly, when the child has a focal deficit that cannot be explained, when the child's progress is not as anticipated, or when the clinical situation is deteriorating slowly, a scan should be obtained. There is no question about the fact that the judicious use of CT scanning in head-injured children has saved many hours of agonizing appraisal and worry in selected cases. No longer do we stand around half the night waiting for angiograms or ventriculograms to suggest to us whether or not there is dangerous pathology present. But it is very important to emphasize that if it seems that a CT scan is necessary, the child already should have been evaluated by a neurosurgeon. Only those experienced in the care of head-injured patients should be making such decisions when time may be of the essence.

Whether or not one has time to obtain a CT scan in a patient who is deteriorating depends on several factors. No neurosurgeon worth his salt would delay for a scan while watching a child previously alert who is becoming unconscious, developing a hemiparesis, a blowing a pupil. That patient required immediate craniotomy, even if carried out in the emergency room. There is no time to lose.

Much more frequently, however, the time-course of deterioration is prolonged, the site of the suspected pathology much less clear. Under such circumstances, it is useful for the surgeon to know exactly where and what the trouble is. If the scanner is close by and not occupied, and if it will take twenty or thirty minutes to prepare the operating room, the CT scan may be of enormous value. Figure 29 is an example of such a situation. This lad of 16 had been injured in a car crash. After a momentary loss of consciousness, he became fully alert. In the emergency room, he showed no neurological abnormalities. However, after about thirty minutes he began to exhibit increasing restlessness, and he complained of headache. His agitation increased. I have learned over the years that when a patient starts becoming agitated following head injury, the physician should become worried. The CT scan showed a large subfrontal extradural hematoma. The clot was removed promptly, and the patient returned to his normal self.

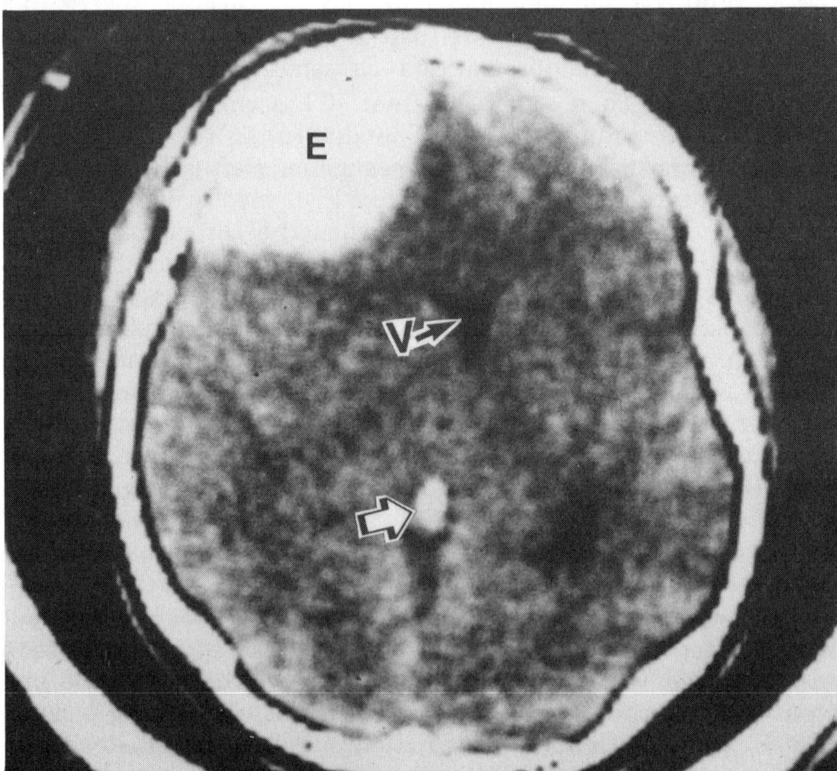

Figure 29. CT scan following head injury.

See text. The subfrontal extradural hematoma is marked by E. The ventricles are shifted to the right, V. The white density marked by the open arrow is the pineal gland. This scan was made on a first-generation machine. Anatomical detail is poor.

Not infrequently there is no surgical mass lesion at all! The CT scanner has significantly reduced the incidence of so-called "woodpecker surgery," the nearly desperate placement of multiple burr holes in the hope — or fear — of finding something.

There is another very useful function of the CT scanner following head injury. Occasionally, patients who have suffered mild, even non-coma producing, injuries will develop symptoms or signs many days, weeks, or months after the event. Intractible headache in the absence of any hard neurological findings is one of the most common of such symptoms. The fact that even "trivial" head injuries can cause the spill of blood into the subarachnoid space is sufficient reason to be concerned about the development of hydrocephalus in such instances. A CT scan quickly decides the issue. Sometimes the headache, very occasionally accompanied by a lateralized neurological deficit, is due to a chronic extracerebral collection of blood or CSF, or to an unsuspected and late-developing intracerebral hematoma. Early discovery of such pathology may spare the patient undue discomfort and risk.

EEG: The electroencephalogram has no place in the early care of the head-injured patient, unless seizures are intractible and surgical pathology has been ruled out. It is reasonable to obtain an EEG if the child has had a post-traumatic seizure, although it is not my practice to do so on that ground alone. If the child was previously epileptic, if seizures recur or are prolonged, or if they are focal, an EEG should be done.

Another indication for doing an EEG is in the child who shows protracted drowsiness in the absence of intracranial pathology on CT scanning, or when intellectual performance is suboptimal. In the latter situation, memory recall is usually the culprit, and temporal lobe dysfunction may be suspected.

Figure 30 is a representative panel from an EEG done on an 11-year-old boy following a concussive head injury. Superficially, he seemed well at discharge, but his school performance two weeks later was below par for him. His examination was normal, he had no headache and no papilledema. The EEG was a surprise. There was a generalized slow wave abnormality coming from his left cerebral hemisphere. Two months later, his school performance was normal, as was his EEG. In this case, the EEG allowed us to evaluate correctly his original injury. In fact, he had suffered a left cerebral contusion, not simply a concussion. Tincture of time corrected the problem.

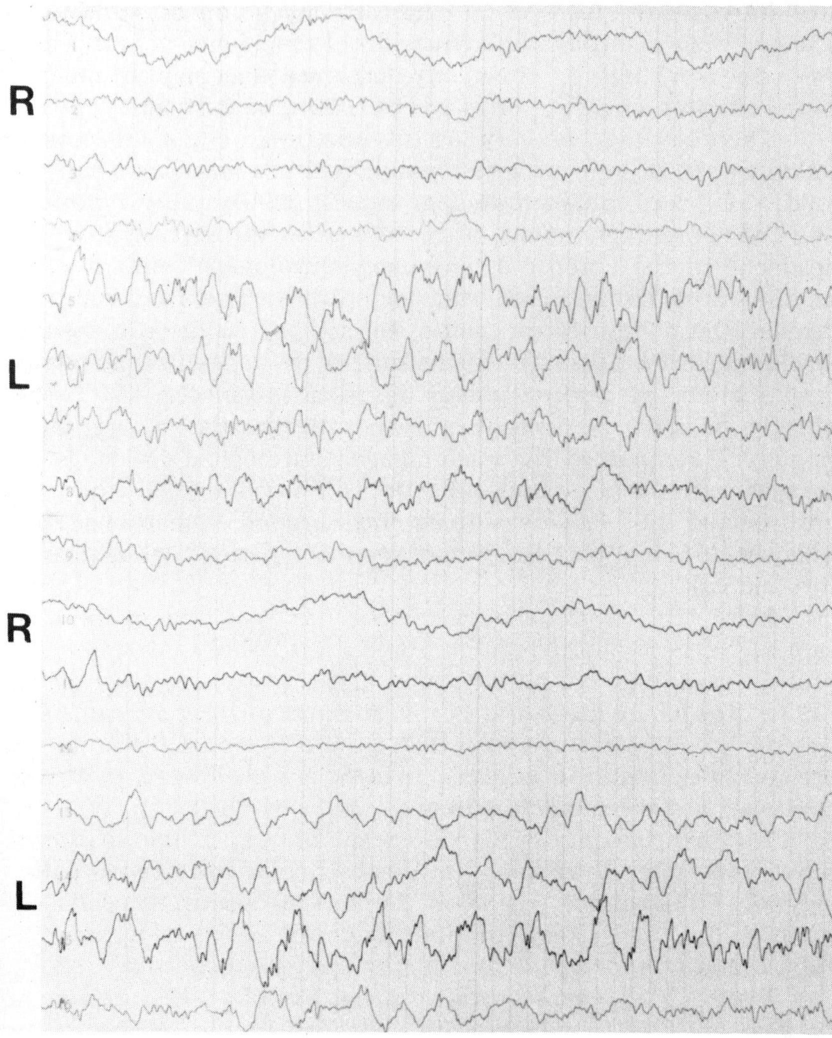

Figure 30. Representative panel of a post-traumatic electroencephalogram.

See text. Lines 1, 2, 3, 4 and 9, 10, 11, 12 are recordings from the right cerebral hemisphere. These rhythms are virtually normal.

It is obvious that the left cerebral recordings are much different. There is a slowing of the wave frequency and a significant increase in wave amplitude. Some of the wave peaks resemble spikes. Such a slow-wave abnormality is common with many types of encephalopathy.

Cerebral Angiograms: Only when CT scanning is unavailable should cerebral angiography be used in the elevation of worrisome cases of head injury. Direct arterial punctures in the neck are seldom justifiable any more, and even the sophisticated catheter techniques carry a small risk — perhaps 1-2% — of arterial wall injury or artery-to-artery embolus. Perhaps the intravenous digital subtraction vascular imaging techniques now in use will prove to be satisfactory as screening procedures in selected patients.

But there is one situation in which careful arterial angiography is important. Not all head injuries in children are quite what they seem initially. Sometimes there is no good reason for the child to have fallen in the first place. Seared into my memory is the example of a 10-year-old boy admitted after a fall from his horse. He was not badly hurt, and he recovered quickly, though he was irritable and complained of severe headache for several days. One month later he had a seizure in bed and rapidly became comatose. He had a ruptured aneurysm (Figure 31) of his distal anterior cerebral artery, and a huge frontal lobe clot. Careful retaking of the initial history suggested that the lad, a very good horse person, had fallen off his mount while the animal was walking. Almost certainly, he fell because his aneurysm bled. Had I recognized the history for what it was at the outset, the aneurysm could have been dealt with easily.

Perhaps I am over-sensitized to the occurrence of vascular events within children's heads. Nevertheless, they occur with sufficient frequency to give one pause. Whenever the history of an apparently straightforward head injury doesn't quite add up, something more must be suspected. Then, a contrast-enhanced CT scan will rule out a tumor or blood-vessel anomaly such as an arteriovenous malformation, but precise arterial angiography is necessary to rule out aneurysms. One of my old surgical mentors told me once: "Things that shouldn't be, ain't."

Lumbar Punctures (LPs): Not only are LP's useless from an information standpoint following head injury, they may be positively dangerous. Even a whack of the head on a cupboard door is likely to cause the spill of a few milliliters of blood into the subarachnoid space. It has been said that as many as 20% of infants born vaginally have blood in the CSF. Small amounts of blood in the CSF are to be expected after even mild head injuries.

The danger arises if one does an LP on a patient who just happens to be developing an intracranial clot. Sudden release of

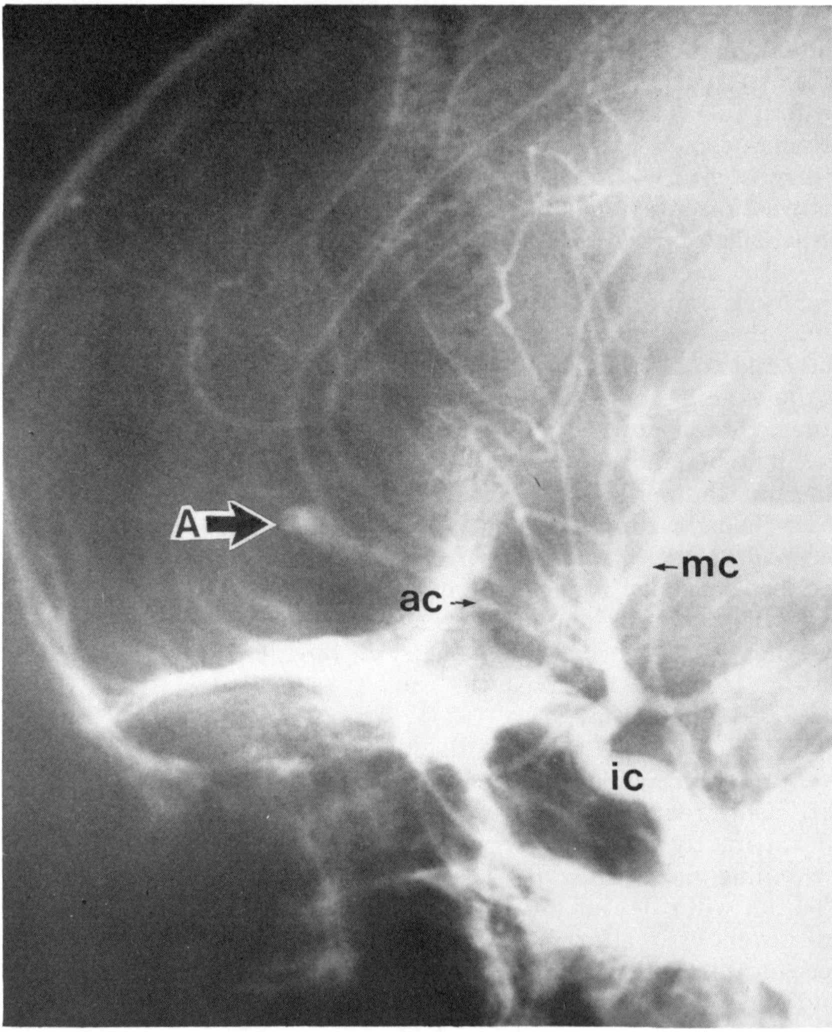

Figure 31. Lateral projection, internal carotid artery angiogram.

See text. ic = internal carotid artery; mc = middle cerebral artery; ac = anterior cerebral artery. The aneurysm — a blow-out of the inner lining of the artery — is shown at A. The wall of an aneurysm lacks the strength of the normal artery wall, and it is liable to rupture, often during episodes when systemic blood pressure is elevated. Blood pouring out of an aneurysm may flood into the subarachnoid space and rip into the brain. ICP may rise catastrophically, and many patients die with the first bleed. Blood in the subarachnoid space may induce severe spasm in nearby arteries, causing cerebral ischemia.

fluid from the spinal theca may change the intracranial pressure balance, encouraging brain tissue to move towards an area of lower pressure. Herniations of cerebellum through the foramen magnum, or of the medial temporal lobes through the tentorial incisura, may result. If such occur, catastrophic deterioration in the patient's status is the rule, and a remedial situation may become hopeless (Figures 21, 22).

Suffice it to say that LPs have **no** place in the early assessment or care of the head-injured patient.

3. SEVERE INJURIES

In Chapter 4, we saw how certain physical forces act to cause varying and unpredictable degrees of brain injury. After the fact, it would be well to have a grade-scoring system that would have predictive and prognostic value. Clinical terms such as stupor, lethargy, obtundation, irritability, even coma, have different meanings for different people. What neurosurgeons needed was a numerical scoring system that would convey from one mind to another a factual assessment of a patient's condition.

a. The Glasgow Coma Scale (GCS)

Bryan Jennett and his colleagues at the University of Glasgow performed for neurosurgeons a great service when they developed the Glasgow Coma Scale. It is not perfect as a coma scoring system, taking all causes of coma into account, but for traumatic coma it has extraordinary value. Now, when I tell another neurosurgeon experienced in trauma that a patient had a six-hour GCS of 6, he and I are on the same wavelength. Instantly, he has an insight into the factual severity of injury, free of such terms as "severe head injury," "light coma," "deep stupor," and so on.

Table 2 is the Glasgow Coma Scale. There are three response categories yielding a total score of 3 through 15. Aesthetically, perhaps, the scoring should range from 0 to 12, but that's the way it is.

There have been criticisms from certain quarters that the GCS is too simple, particularly that it ignores brain stem reflexes. We shall comment upon this matter shortly. For traumatic coma, the overriding advantages of the GCS are as follows:

1. It is simple to perform, takes little time, hence can be repeated frequently;

TABLE 2 **GLASGOW COMA SCALE**

Score	Response Category		
	MOTOR	VERBAL	EYE OPENING
6	Obeys	——	——
5	Localizes	Oriented	——
4	Normal Flexor (Good Withdrawal)	Confused	Spontaneously
3	Abnormal Flexor (Purposeless, Random)	Inappropriate, But Says Words	To Sound
2	Extensor (Decerebrate)	Incomprehensible, But Utters Sounds	To Pain
1	Nil	Nil	Nil

NOTE: RECORD BEST RESPONSE, FROM BEST SIDE.
ANY FALL-OFF IN NUMERICAL SCORE IS A DANGER SIGN.

2. The responses are unequivocal, hence the total score is representative of reality;
3. Paramedicals learn the system quickly and can perform it with accuracy;
4. It is reproducible from one examiner to another;
5. It has predictive value.

The GCS should be an integral part of the finger-tip knowledge and capacity of everyone who deals with traumatic coma. A score established immediately following injury becomes the bench-mark of the clinical course of the patient. You will note from the table that a rising score indicates improvement, one that is falling signals deterioration.

Sometimes the respiratory efficiency of the patient is compromised because of the degree of brain injury, facial and neck injury, or chest trauma. In such circumstances it may be necessary to insert an endotracheal tube. Obviously, that event obviates the middle response category. The examiner then inserts the letter T as the middle score. It is best always to use the format 6–5–4 for scoring. A patient with an endotracheal tube might have a score of 4–T–2. To any neurosurgeon experienced in trauma, such a score will have validity.

Very occasionally, both eyes become swollen shut very early on. Then, the letter S is inserted in the third column. Even if both the Verbal and Eye Opening categories are compromised by the letters T and S, the Motor Response category will yield very useful information.

Those of us with extensive experience with the GCS in traumatic coma have little patience with the criticisms of the scale. It may seem strange that the GCS ignores brain stem reflexes, but the reasons are quite simple. First, the brain stem reflexes reflect pathology or lack thereof at different levels of the brain stem. For example, the pupillary responses correspond to the midbrain; corneal reflexes reflect mid-pontine function; eye movements in response to warm or cold water irrigation of the ear canals (caloric responses), as well as the "doll's-eyes" reflexes, correlate with pontine and upper medulla function. Each reflex would be recorded separately, as a 1 or 2 (nil or present) response. That would make 7 response categories.

Second, motor responses reflect brain stem levels very well. Stereotyped extensor motor responses correspond to pontine/lower midbrain dysfunction; stereotyped flexor responses indicate a high midbrain/diencephalon level. The same reasoning applies to criticisms relating to omission of the breathing patterns. The purpose of the GCS is to provide reliable, reproducible information as simply as possible, information that does, in fact, indicate what is happening to the patient.

Finally, the GCS has predictive value. For example, in the absence of intoxication or hypothermia, I have never seen an adult patient recover completely if his post-traumatic GCS six hours following injury was less than 6. You will note that I specified "adult." With children, I cannot be so dogmatic; even so, recovery can be a relative term, as we shall see in Chapter 6.

Having said all of that, there are two codacils. (1) The GCS is difficult to apply to infants, and modifications are available. All they really demand is a familiarity with infant development patterns and age-norm levels. (2) It is extremely useful, when practicable, for the initial examiner to record pupillary responses as a separate notation. Even here, problems arise. A blow on or near an orbit may cause a "traumatic mydriasis," a pupil paralysed at full dilation by the local trauma itself.

As a final caveat regarding brain stem reflexes, the "doll's-eye" reflex, a maneuver requiring rotation of the head on the neck, must not be done if the integrity of the cervical spine is in doubt.

In general, any patient whose GCS is 8 or less several minutes following trauma has sustained a very serious, potentially lethal head injury. And it cannot be emphasized too strongly that any GCS score that is falling also indicates a potentially lethal situation.

b. Intracranial Pressure (ICP) Monitoring

Table 3 is an alorgithm of my triage routine for severely head-injured patients. As a rule, any patient whose GCS is 8 or less at examination in the emergency room, or whose GCS score is falling, fits into this scheme.

Not all patients who must be rushed off to the operating room end up with an ICP monitor post-operatively. This is particularly so for patients with extradural hematomas. Such patients, if intercepted in time, will do very well. Often they are awake with minimal findings within a few hours of operation. To insert an ICP monitor in such patients would be meddlesome.

Intracranial pressure monitoring has been very useful to clinicians in the understanding of the dynamics of severe brain injury. Years ago, we might examine a patient shortly following injury and find that he was showing neurogenic hyperventilation, abnormal flexor motor responses, normal brain stem reflexes, groaning to pain, and no eye opening (GCS of 3-2-1=7). His fundi would be normal. Such a patient we would classify as a "primary brain stem injury, normal ICP." The CT scan has shown us that almost always such patients have diffuse brain injury, with focal or widespread edema and, often, small parenchymal hemorrhages especially at the base of the frontal and temporal lobes. So much

TABLE 3

TRIAGE OF SEVERE HEAD INJURY

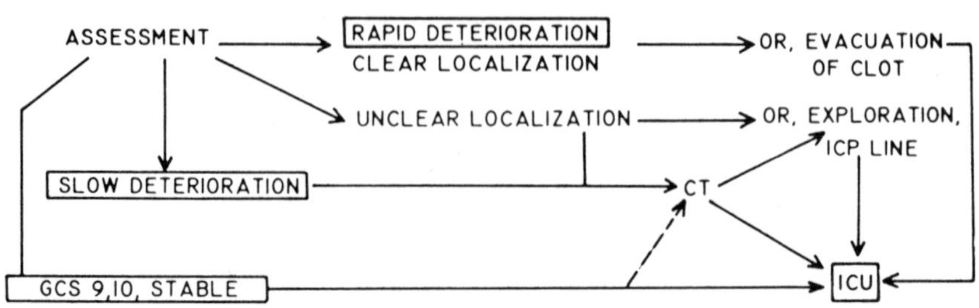

for the frequency of primary brain stem injuries. ICP monitoring has made us aware that this same patient usually has mildly to severely raised ICP, frequently with superimposed ICP spikes with maximum mean ICP reaching levels of 40 or 50 torr, even higher, for several seconds, even minutes. Figure 18 is an ICP record from just such a patient. Sometimes the ICP base line is dangerously high, 30 or 40 torr, without ICP spike phenomena. Our clinical methods for estimating ICP are not very reliable.

Not infrequently, a severely-injured patient will have episodes spontaneously of extensor posturing — decerebrate rigidity. With an ICP trace running, it is possible to time the onset of the extensor "fit" with respect to an intracranial pressure wave, if such are occurring. When they are associated — more than half of the time, in my experience — almost always the ICP begins to rise before the decerebrate spasm commences, indicating that the ICP wave is the probable causal antecedent of the extensor episode, not vice versa.

From ICP monitoring, we have been able to appreciate graphically the effect of various agents and maneuvers upon ICP. Some of these effects are shown in Figure 32. Osmotic agents take twenty or thirty minutes to exert full effect upon ICP, whereas intravenous boluses of such things as thiopental, alpha-thesin and lidocaine will induce a sudden drop in ICP. Vigorous hyperventilation will do the same, in most individuals.

The pattern of ICP that a patient shows has some predictive value. All of us engaged in intensive monitoring of severely head-injured patients agree that those patients whose ICPs stay high despite all therapeutic measures (30 torr or greater) have a very poor outcome, universally. What is not yet proven is whether or not control of ICP to levels of 20 or 25 torr or less has any significant bearing upon outcome. Further, there are some patients whose ICPs never rise above normal who do very badly. Logically, one might assume that if unremittingly high ICP is strongly associated with a lethal or vegetative outcome, control of ICP to levels where cerebral perfusion pressure (CPP) always remains above 50 torr should be beneficial. It is true that for patients whose ICPs are easily controlled or remain below 20 without therapy, prognosis is much better. Unfortunately, to this date we simply cannot prove that our therapeutic efforts are of significant value.

My own preference for ICP monitoring technique is the placement of a fine catheter in the lateral ventricle. Figure 33 illus-

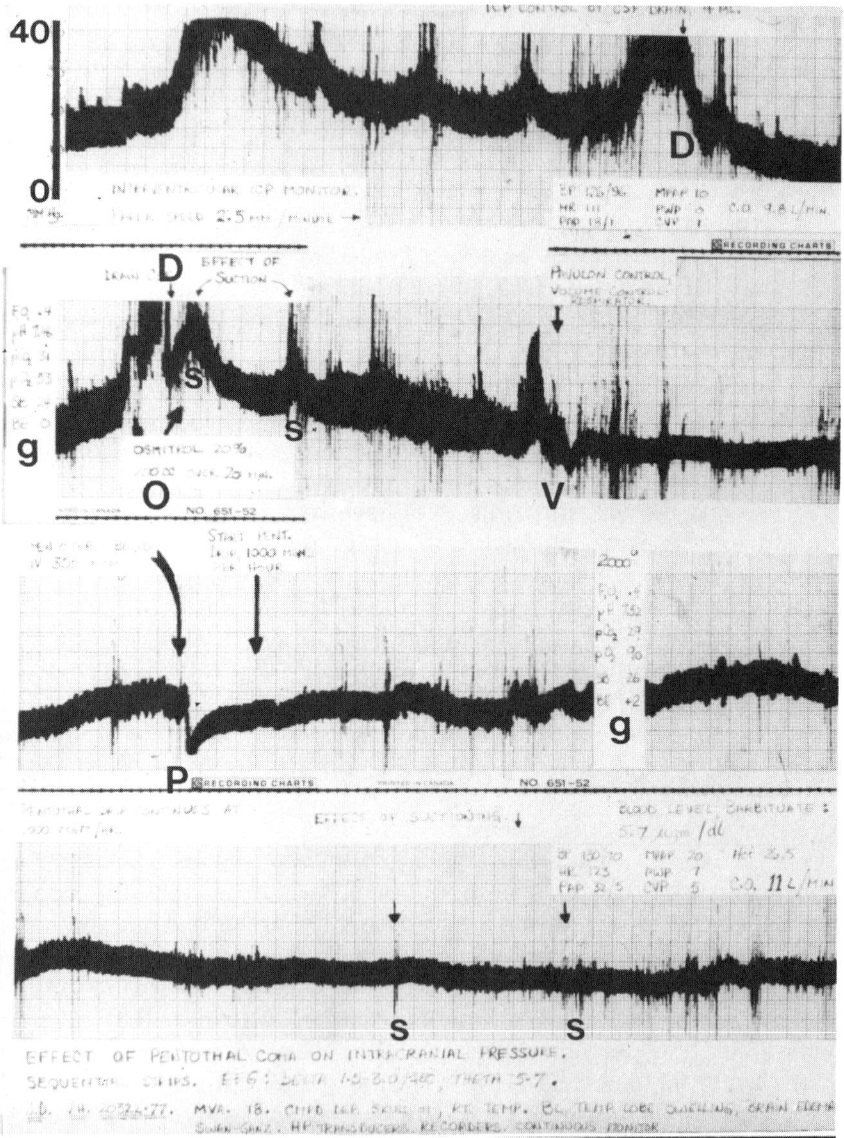
40
0
D
D
EFFECT OF SUCTION
S
S
g
O
V
OSMITROL 20%
NO. 651-52
RECORDING CHARTS
START PENT.
P
g
NO. 651-52
EFFECT OF SUCTIONING
S
S
EFFECT OF PENTOTHAL COMA ON INTRACRANIAL PRESSURE.
SEQUENTIAL STRIPS.

Figure 32. Continuous ICP recording following trauma, intraventricular catheter.

The paper speed is 2.5 mm per minute, each large square representing two minutes real time. Pressure values in torr (mm Hg). Vertical strips marked "g" are blood gas values. Events D mark CSF volume drainage to control ICP. Events marked s show ICP responses to endotracheal suction.

At 0 on second line, an intravenous 20% solution of mannitol was begun. A gradual fall in ICP is apparent over the next 30 minutes, ending in another sharp elevation of ICP during suctioning. At V, the patient's respirations were brought under control of a ventilator by means of a pavulon (a paralysing drug) drip.

At P, third line, a 350 mgm bolus of sodium pentothal was given intravenously. Note the sharp, sudden drop in ICP, with slow rise over seven minutes. At the second arrow, line 3, a pentothal continuous drip was instituted. Within an hour, control of ICP is very steady. Note that the ICP response to suctioning is abolished, on bottom line.

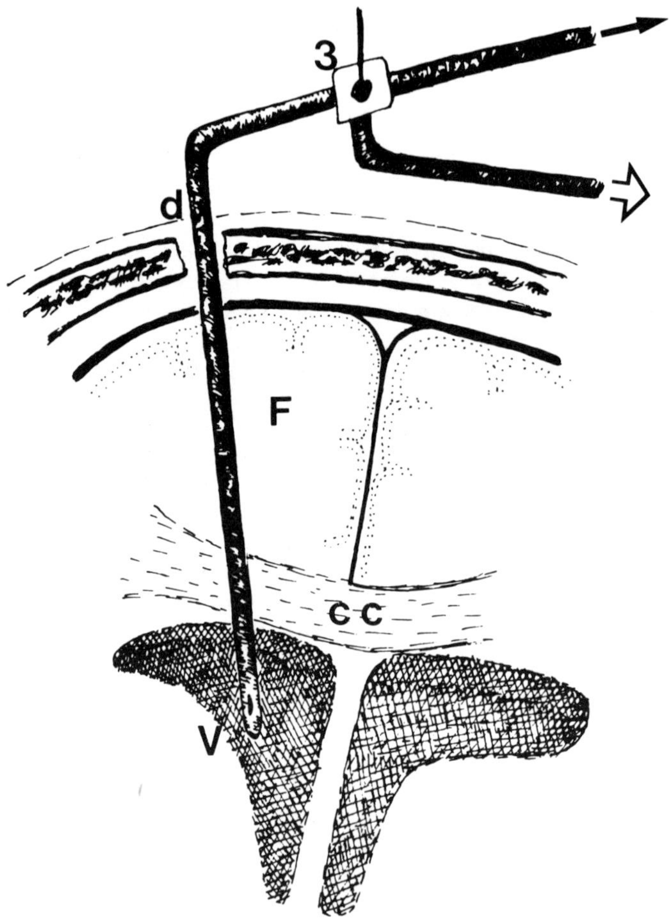

Figure 33. Principle of ICP monitoring using ventricular catheter.

The ventricular catheter enters the cranium through a twist-drill hole, (d). It traverses the frontal lobe (F), the corpus callosum (cc) to enter the lateral ventricle (V). Externally, the catheter is connnected to a 3-way stop-clock (3), hence to a pressure transducer (small arrow) for ICP measurement, or to a drainage bag (open arrow) for fluid drainage to help control ICP.

trates the principles. The ventricle is close to the center of the head, hence, it is likely to reflect accurately and very early changes in ICP. An outlet from the CSF-filled catheter proximal to the pressure transducer serves as a drain for CSF, thereby reducing intracranial volume, hence ICP.

Several devices are available for monitoring ICP from the brain surface. The principal advantages of such subdurally — or epidurally — placed devices are (1) greater ease of placement — sometimes it is very difficult or impossible to hit a very small ventricle; (2) greater safety — occasionally the attempt to place a catheter in the ventricle is the cause of an intracerebral hemorrhage; (3) less risk of infection — but with proper placement and subcutaneous tunneling of the ventricular catheter, and strict aseptic care, the risk of introducing infection into the ventricles with the catheter technique should be less than 1%.

Sometimes our therapeutic efforts to lower ICP — especially when barbiturates are in use — result in a critical lowering of CPP. At that point, one is defeating an originally good intention. All too often, in very badly injured patients, we end up infusing agents in one arm that not only lower ICP but mean arterial pressure as well, and an agent such as dopamine in the other arm in order to shore up the mean arterial pressure. My experience is that such a situation is hopeless; the ICU staff at my place calls this combination of pharmacologies "embalming fluid."

There are two other caveats relating to ICP monitoring that deserve brief mention. (1) Recent animal work in our laboratories indicates that when the blood-brain barrier is disrupted, as it often is at least focally in trauma, too high a CPP promotes more cerebral edema by hydrostatically driving fluid into the brain. Thus, in head injury, there is both a critical lower *and higher* limit for CPP. (2) Not infrequently, drugs used to control ICP or to keep a patient in good synchronization with a respirator result in complete loss of peripheral motor responses and brain stem reflexes. Then, one must rely upon the ICP value and judicious use of repeat CT scanning to monitor intracranial pathology. Obviously, such care can be carried out only in well-equipped units.

On balance, ICP monitoring is a very useful adjunct to the care of the severely head-injured patient. With it, we have a much clearer picture of what is going on inside the head. And one certainly feels better if the ICP is remaining close to normal values.

Still, it is not the magic wand for producing better results that some have implied.

c. The Art of Observation

I believe that it was Jonathan Swift who stated that "observation is the art of seeing things not yet visible." Maybe it wasn't, but it should have been.

Neurosurgeons depend to a much greater extent than often they will admit upon the perspicacity and common sense of the nurses trained in the art of close observation of dangerously ill or injured patients. Only time and repetition of observational techniques, and a willing and absorptive mind, can turn a green observer into a skilled one. To paraphrase old Euclid, "there is no royal road to neurological competence."

Historically, the work sheet of the neurosurgical observer has been something commonly entitled "Neurological Observation Record," or some such thing. Of course, these records are very important, but only if the assessments are done with appropriate frequency. Figure 34 is the form in use in our neurosurgical observation units. In conjunction with an ICP tracing, and when a simultaneous record is kept of cerebral perfusion pressure, such a form recorded frequently enough, is of enormous value. When patients are sick enough to require the use of an "NOR" or "NSR" or whatever it is called, they deserve continuous care. Such orders as "NSR four-hourly," often written by physicians, are laughable. Even the very common "NSR hourly" is valueless if constant observation is not provided. We have noted previously how a CPP reduced below a critical level for more than two or three *minutes* may be lethal to brain function. Many a patient has died or become irreversibly damaged during the intervals of a carefully recorded observation sheet. Every person entrusted with the care of patients with severe head injury — or any neurological disorder involving abnormalities of ICV and ICP, for that matter — must remember constantly that for such patients, time equates with brain function. Prompt reporting of any deleterious change in neurological function is mandatory.

After a time, skilled and experienced observers acquire a "sixth sense" about patients' conditions. These are the people who have achieved the art of observation. A miniscule drop in the level of alertness or conscious state; a subtle change in the breathing pattern; the onset of restlessness often heralded by a tendency to

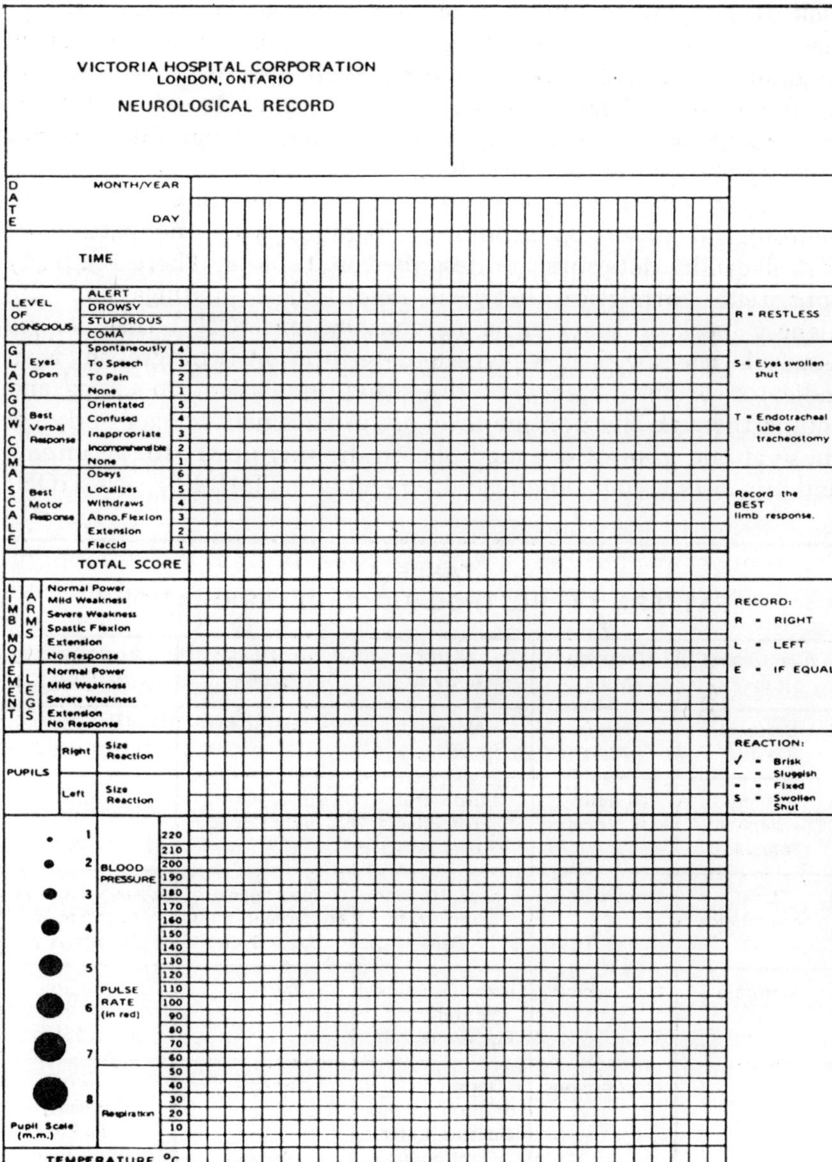

VICTORIA HOSPITAL CORPORATION
LONDON, ONTARIO
NEUROLOGICAL RECORD

DATE — MONTH/YEAR — DAY

TIME

LEVEL OF CONSCIOUS: ALERT; DROWSY; STUPOROUS; COMA — R = RESTLESS

GLASGOW COMA SCALE

Eyes Open: Spontaneously 4; To Speech 3; To Pain 2; None 1 — S = Eyes swollen shut

Best Verbal Response: Orientated 5; Confused 4; Inappropriate 3; Incomprehensible 2; None 1 — T = Endotracheal tube or tracheostomy

Best Motor Response: Obeys 6; Localizes 5; Withdraws 4; Abno.Flexion 3; Extension 2; Flaccid 1 — Record the BEST limb response.

TOTAL SCORE

LIMB MOVEMENT

ARMS: Normal Power; Mild Weakness; Severe Weakness; Spastic Flexion; Extension; No Response

LEGS: Normal Power; Mild Weakness; Severe Weakness; Extension; No Response

RECORD: R = RIGHT; L = LEFT; E = IF EQUAL

PUPILS: Right — Size, Reaction; Left — Size, Reaction

REACTION: ✓ = Brisk; — = Sluggish; • = Fixed; S = Swollen Shut

Pupil Scale (m.m.): 1, 2, 3, 4, 5, 6, 7, 8

BLOOD PRESSURE; PULSE RATE (in red): 220, 210, 200, 190, 180, 170, 160, 150, 140, 130, 120, 110, 100, 90, 80, 70, 60, 50, 40

Respiration: 30, 20, 10

TEMPERATURE °C

Figure 34. NSR record.

Note that the Glasgow Coma Scale is incorporated into the record. All important neurological and cardiopulmonary parameters should be readily visible on a single sheet. Such record sheets are very useful in showing trends in the patient's condition.

pick at bedclothes, intravenous lines, or bandages; such things alert the observer to impending trouble long before a pupil begins to dilate or a hemiparesis appears. Such was the case with the patient whose CT has been described in Figure 29. That lad owes his well-being to a very sharp nurse whose mind and observational skills were tuned in to subtle things.

As an aid to assessment of the level of neurological function, neurological observers should be familiar with the pattern of rostral-caudal deterioration described in Table 4. There is a fairly consistent correlation between neurological findings and the highest level of the central nervous system (CNS) that can be assessed. The speed at which the deterioration is progressing is an indicator of the urgency of the situation. Patients reaching and sliding through the pontine level are in imminent danger of dying; those at the level of the medulla, on the way down, for all intents and purposes are already dead. Remember—TIME IS FUNCTION!

TABLE 4
PATTERN OF ROSTROCAUDAL DETERIORATION

Functioning Level	*Conscious State*	*Motor Activity*	*Breathing Pattern*	*Brain Stem Reflexes*
Cerebral Cortex	Normal Alert	Normal ± Focal Deficit	Normal	Normal
High Diencephalon (Thalamus)	Rousable May Vocalize	Purposeful, Protective ± Focal Deficit	Usually Normal Early Cyclic	Normal
Low Diencephalon	Unconscious	Flexor, Random Withdraw to Pain	Neurogenic Hyperventilation Early Cyclic	Usually Normal Autonomic Overactivity
Midbrain	Unconscious	Flexor, Occasional Extensor, Posture to Pain	Cyclical	Fixed Pupils
Pons	Unconscious	Extensor, to Pain or Spontaneous Spasms, Later, Continuous	Apneustic Ataxic	Loss of Corneals, Doll's Eyes Pupils Tiny or Dilated
Medulla	Unconscious	Flaccid	Agonal	Loss of Cardio-Respiratory Control

d. Child Abuse

Of all the acts perpetrated by one human upon another, none is as foul, as dispicable, as the intentional injury of a child by its parent or guardian. Physical child abuse is endemic in western European and North American society, virtually unheard of in oriental, polynesian, Indian, and primitive cultures. Precise figures for incidence in North America are unavailable, as many instances go undetected. It is estimated that 2,500 cases of child abuse occur yearly in the province of Ontario, population 8.5 million. Between 10 and 25% of these come to attention, and of that number, 20 to 30% will be permanently damaged or will die. Many will have been abused previously.

It has been my sorry lot to care for children whose heads have been crushed by a boot, split open by being swung against a wall or door frame, whose brains have been contused by direct blows, whose bodies have been immersed in scalding hot water or used as ash trays for butting cigarettes. It is difficult to believe such wanton cruelty, but it happens as a matter of course. Figure 35 is an example of an abused infant following craniotomy for removal of a subdural hematoma. Many bruises, of differing ages, are visible on the child's body.

The substrate from which horrors emanate commonly is that of young, immature parents, one or both of whom have little or no impulse control. Too often, the parents are unemployed, under substantial stress financially and in interpersonal relations. The incidents of abuse occur frequently when only one parent or guardian is home.

To be fair, sometimes it is simply a matter of a loving parent not realizing how fragile an infant really is. Even the shaking of a baby with unsupported head is quite sufficient to cause an acute subdural bleed. I well recall one father whose habit it was to toss his son up into the air, catching him to the giggling delight of the infant. One day he missed. He was careless, not intentionally cruel, but the result for the child was just as unpleasant.

Virtually every legal jurisdiction now has mandatory reporting statues for suspected child abuse. In every such case, the reporting party is protected from legal retribution should the situation prove otherwise. Unfortunately, not always do the child protection agencies provide sufficient protection for the child later on, and repeat incidents of child abuse are all too common.

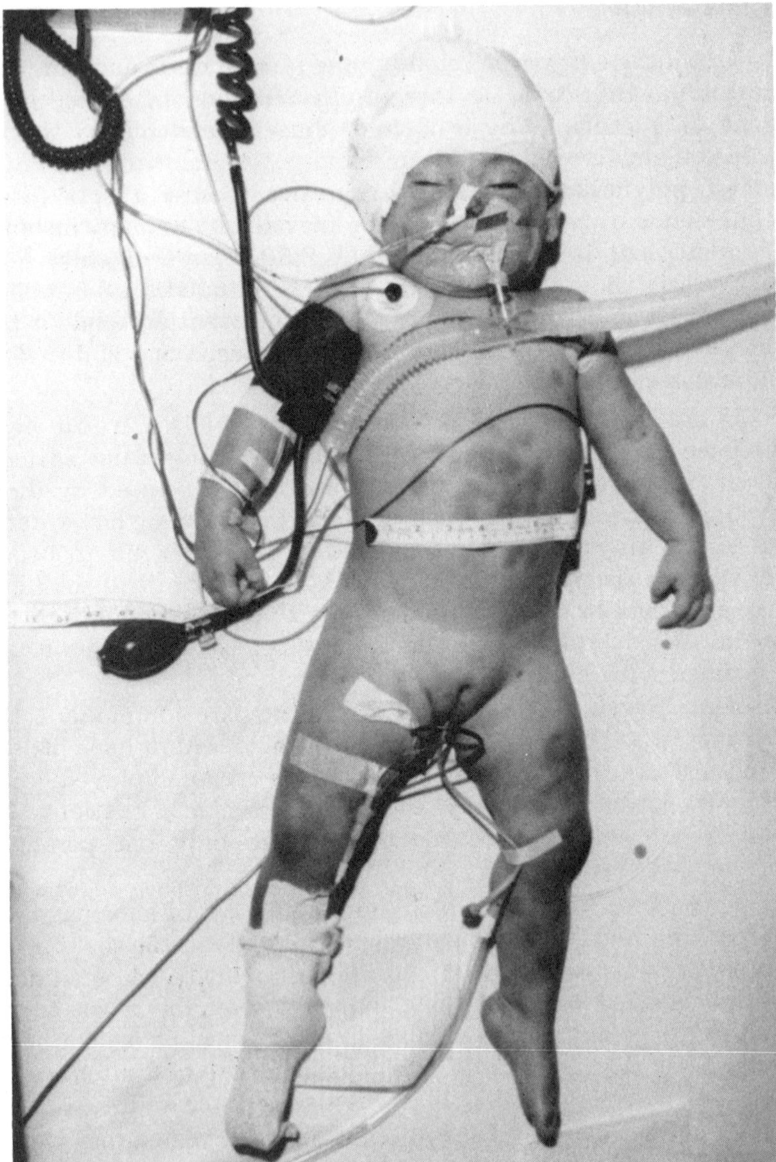

Figure 35. An abused child.

This photograph was taken following craniotomy. Note the facial swelling and bruising, and the bruises on arms, chest, abdomen, and legs. This baby sustained tremendous right cerebral contusion and swelling after being swung by the feet against a wall. She survived only a few days.

I can smell it when a child has been abused. The injury is incompatible with the history; the history is inconsistent; there are unexplained bruises some place; there is a pattern that becomes unmistakable. Total body x-rays are imperative; quite often an old, healed, and previously unreported fracture will turn up.

Most children's centers have developed a "Child Abuse Team," consisting of a supervisory physician and social workers skilled in ferreting out and pinpointing the causative factors. Many of the responsible adults can be rehabilitated, some cannot; therein lies the overriding challenge of the team. Children should be with their parents, if it is safe, but their protection is the prime imperative.

e. The Outcome From Severe Head Injury

It is unlikely that anyone recovers completely from any head injury if their GCS, in the absence of intoxication, hypothermia or hypovolemic shock, six hours after injury remains 9 or 10 or below. The rationale for this statement will be more obvious from the discussion in Chapter 6.

It is, unfortunately, very difficult to compare data from different centers. The patient mix often is non-comparable. Until Glasgow Coma Scale (GCS) values came into common use, it was even hard to be sure what another reporter really meant by severe injury. Now, at least, we have some basis for comparison.

In a very significant report from the Ranchos Los Amigos children's head injury rehabilitation service published in 1980, some very sobering figures were presented. All of the children and adolescents had survived a period of traumatic coma of at least 24 hours — the authors could not use the GCS as original assessments had not consistently used the scale — durations of coma ranging from over 24 hours to more than 6 weeks. It is safe to assume that all the patients had GCS values of 10 or less at the 24 hour mark. Forty-four percent had required emergency neurosurgical procedures.

Of this cohort, 73% regained independent ambulatory and self-care status by one year, 10% were partially, and 17% were totally dependent. Eight percent remained comatose. Only 10% had a normal motor examination one year following injury, and of that group, 72% were deficient in intellectual functioning; conversely, 28% scored within the normal IQ range.

Even that figure is misleading, for it is unlikely that many of the tested subjects had had previous neuropsychological testing with which to compare. A child scoring at 130 pre-trauma may still fit into the normal range with a post-traumatic score of 95, but his intellectual potential has been very significantly reduced.

Twenty-six percent of this group had early seizures, 9% had late seizures. The incidence of recurrent seizures — epilepsy — was not stated.

Nineteen of the original cohort died after admission to the rehabilitation center (5.5%), all from the severely damaged group.

Such data are all the more startling when you recall that they apply to the *survivors* of the original head-injured patients. In my personal experience, the majority of severely head-injured patients have been within, or have been struck by, a motor vehicle. Many sustained multiple-organ trauma. Of 109 patients whose GCS in the emergency room was 9 or less, 53 died, (49%). In fairness, 15 of these were essentially brain-dead upon arrival, leaving 38 who died within hours to ten days of admission (40% of 94). Twenty of those 38 deaths occurred in children with severe multiple-organ injury. These victims were cared for in an extremely active critical care/trauma unit, so their deaths cannot be ascribed to lack of level I care, as outlined by the American College of Surgeons.

There is one recent report from the Philadelphia Children's Hospital that had only a 6% acute mortality in head-injured patients. No other series has approached that admirable statistic but the patient mix ratios very probably play a large part in the discrepancies. The important point is that major blunt impact trauma combined with head injury in young people is a lethal business, and that the number that recover completely, physically and mentally, is discouragingly small. At this juncture, much clinical effort is being directed to the improvement of such results. Whether significant improvement in the rate of return to full independent physical activity *and* pre-traumatic intellect will occur remains to be seen, but we must try. Twenty-five thousand dead and disabled young people from head injury, each year, in the United States alone, is an epidemic of carnage and loss of human potential that shames us all.

4. ASSOCIATED INJURIES

We have made it quite clear at various points in our discourse that head injury frequently occurs in association with trauma to other areas of the body and organ systems. We have emphasized that hypovolemic shock may have extremely deleterious effects upon the brain, and that multiple-organ injury may have lethal consequences. We have noted that trauma-induced abnormalities in water and electrolyte balance and metabolism can make the care of these patients complex and difficult. Still, there are certain injuries that deserve special emphasis. We shall look at these in this section.

a. Spinal Injury

Falls and major blunt injury in particular have an inordinate association with injuries to the spinal column. It is critical that every person who has anything to do with the care and handling of patients unconscious from trauma be aware of this fact constantly. What a tragedy it is when a patient with an unstable spine but no spinal cord damage is rendered para- or quadriplegic by improper handling at the scene of the accident, or in the emergency room.

Of course, a patient in coma will not respond to inquiries regarding motor power or sensation or sites of pain in the back or neck. When the injury is such that spinal column damage reasonably may have occurred, spinal cord injury precautions are mandatory. This means that the victim is to be moved without allowing *any* relative motion — flexion, extension, rotation — between the head and neck or any part of the spine and another. If the patient is face down, a folded towel or a cervical collar should be wrapped around the neck first, then the patient should be turned as a unit. Transfers of the patient from one stretcher or whatever to another must be minimized. During transport, the neck is to be supported by a cervical collar that maintains immobility. If such a patient requires endotracheal intubation, extreme care must be used. The result of sudden, sharp extension of the head by a panicky attendant trying to insert the tube can be catastrophic for the cervical spinal cord.

Usually, it is possible to ascertain that the cord already has been damaged, even in an unconscious patient. If the level of coma is such that limb motor responses should occur with peripheral stimulation, the absence of such responses is presumptive evidence for spinal cord injury. For example, a patient unresponsive to voice, with no eye opening and no vocalization, but with briskly reactive pupils and a normal or high brain stem level breathing pattern, would be expected to show *at least* an extensor limb response to strong cutaneous stimulation. If such does not occur in any limb, one must worry about a cervical cord injury. If a motor response occurs in the arms but not the legs, one thinks of a thoracic cord injury.

Unconscious patients usually will demonstrate the phenomenon of pupillary dilatation in response to peripheral painful stimulation. This test may be useful in establishing an approximate level of spinal cord injury. Many hospitals now are equipped to carry out spinal cord assessment by multiple modality evoked cortical responses. For instance, the quality and rate of transmission of peripheral cutaneous stimuli up the spinal cord to the brain can be measured accurately by appropriate instruments. The stimulus is applied by a set of electrodes on the skin, and the response discharge picked up from scalp electrodes. The same sort of measurements can be made for the auditory and visual systems.

The more proximally (cranially) the spinal cord is injured, the more likely is the victim to demonstrate the "sympathectomy effect." Stimulation of the sympathetic nervous systems (SNS) — part of the autonomic ("automatic") central nervous system — causes an increase in the tone in blood vessels, an increase in heart rate, increased sweating, piloerection, and a major part of the complex micturition reflex. Sympathetic nervous system outflow to the body occurs through the thoracic spinal cord. Thus, injury to the cervical cord causes a sudden loss of all SNS to the periphery. The result is a slow heart rate (bradycardia); warm, dry skin due to vasodilatation throughout the skin and lack of sweating; low blood pressure, due to pooling of blood in muscle, skin, and viscera; urine retention; priapism (reflex erection). Inexperienced observers may mistake the hypotension for a sign of internal bleeding; in fact, the entire picture is a sure sign of spinal cord injury.

There is a caveat worth remembering in this context, though. Free blood in the peritoneal cavity is very irritating, and induces a reflex contraction of the abdominal wall muscles. If the spinal cord is damaged, this warning sign of intra-abdominal bleeding will not be seen.

Obviously, when spinal cord damage is suspected, spinal x-rays are required. When coma is due to falls or blunt impact, it is my practice to obtain films of the cervical spine, at the very least. The cervical spine is vulnerable to damage, whenever hyperflexion or hyperextension of the head on the neck may have occurred. It is essential that the x-rays show all levels of the vertebral column to the junction of the seventh cervical and first thoracic vertebrae. All due precautions in moving the patient must be observed until one is certain that the spine is intact.

Figure 36 is a lateral cervical spine x-ray from a 15-month-old girl. She had been thrown about inside a car during a collision, was momentarily unconscious. She was felt to be fine when examined in an emergency room, and was sent home. Within a few days, she was holding her head stiffly forward on her neck, had neck discomfort, and refused to walk. Two weeks later, the spine film showed a fracture at the base of the odontoid process of the second cervical vertebral body, with dislocation anteriorly of C1 upon C2, the dislocation carrying the odontoid process forward, as well. The fracture was firmly stuck in its abnormal position by this time. Removal of the posterior arch of C1 (the atlas) relieved the child's neck pain, and she took up walking once again, with a vengeance.

Usually it requires much greater force to disrupt the integrity of the thoracic or lumbar spines than it does the cervical. Events such as long falls onto the back or rump and violent vehicular impacts are the usual culprits. The buttressing effects of the rib-cage, the more massive bony construction, the larger paraspinal muscles, and the orientation of the intervertebral articular facets, are the protective factors. A few moments study of a demonstration spine will reinforce your appreciation of these factors.

In summary, the specter of spinal cord injury must be remembered and, if possible, averted by everyone involved in caring for head-injured patients.

b. Chest Wall and Lung Injury

We mentioned this association briefly in Chapter 4. Chest wall injury may interfere with efficient gas exchange in the lungs, threatening the damaged brain with the extra problem of hypoxia. Fractured ribs may puncture the lung, releasing air into the pleural cavity and reducing functional lung volume. An open chest wound may allow air to be sucked into the chest during inspiration.

Lung injury may arise from blunt impact, from laceration by a rib or perforating object, or from aspirated blood, vomitus, or foreign material. The last mentioned situation causes consolidation of some lung volume and severe inflammation of large and small bronchial tubes.

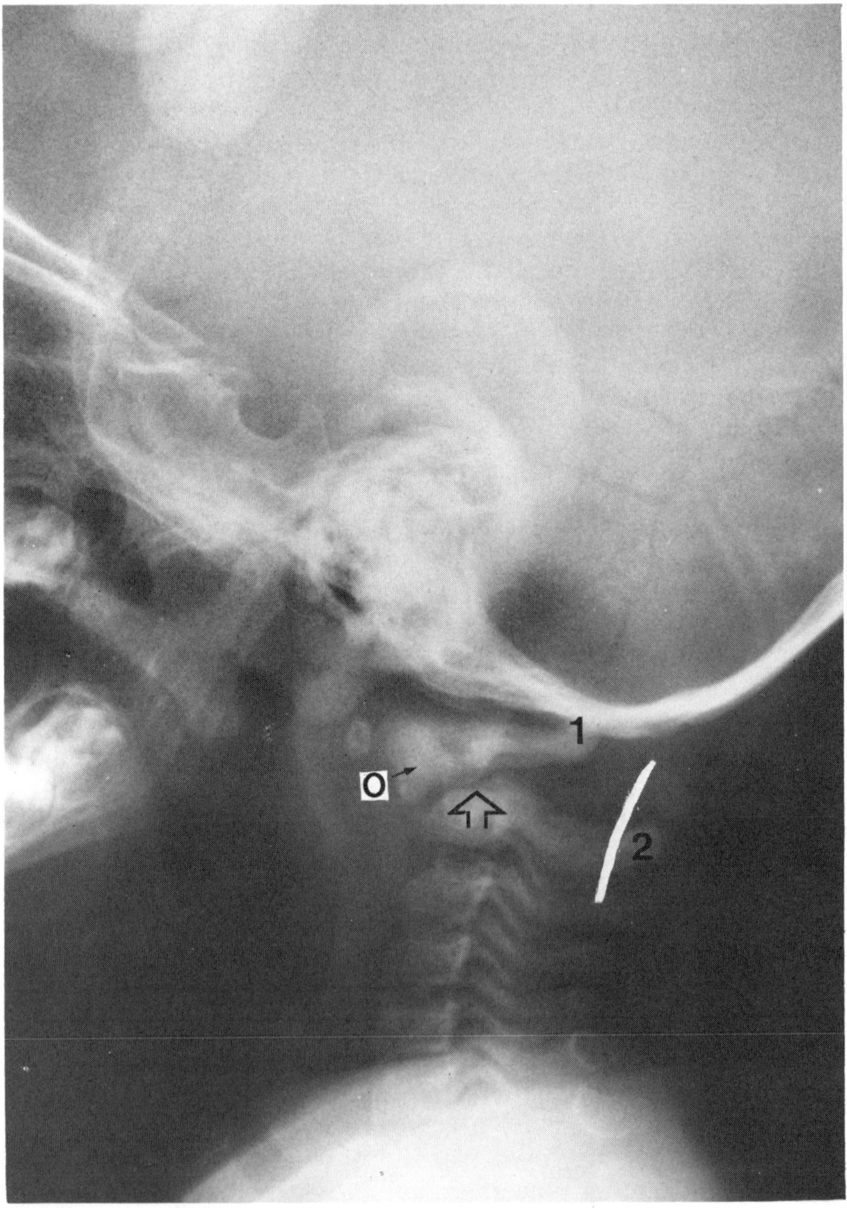
1
O
2

Figure 36. Fracture of odontoid process with forward displacement of first cervical vertebra and odontoid.

See text. "o" marks odontoid process. It should sit directly above open arrow. The posterior rim of C1 (marked by 1) is displaced anteriorly and superiorly, constricting the spinal canal at this level. 1 should sit on or just behind the white line.

Note that this particular radiograph is inadequate for visualization of the lower cervical spine. The body of C7 is not visible.

To date, no means is known of inducing damaged nerve fibres in the brain or spinal cord to regenerate themselves. If a fracture-dislocation of the spine causes interruption of the physical integrity of nerve fibres, no nerve impulses will pass up or down beyond that point, ever again. Damage to the spinal cord below the first thoracic vertebral level causes paraplegia, paralysis of the legs and rectal and urinary sphincters, and varying degrees of paralysis of the chest-wall muscles of respiration. If the level of damage is higher, the following muscle groups are added to the litany, in increasing severity of quadriplegia:

C8 - T1 — muscles of the hands
C7 - C8 — muscles of forearms, triceps
C6 - C7 — upper arms
C5 - C6 — shoulder girdle
C1 - C5 — diaphragm (total respiratory paralysis)

The end result for the brain is the same, whether it arises from inadequate ventilation of sufficient lung tissue or imperfect gas exchange at the alveoli-capillary interface: hypoxia. I look upon the combination of head and chest injury as more than just additive insults. It is a tragedy when a patient with a relatively mild brain injury is rendered brain-dead because the chest injury was not handled promptly and adequately.

Patients with significant chest wall or lung injury usually deserve endotracheal intubation. Very often, their ICV-ICP relationship is teetering on the brink of runaway ICP. The very act of intubation, and the suctioning and re-positioning of endotracheal tubes, commonly induce very high amplitude ICP waves, if precautions are not taken. We have found it advantageous to paralyse the patient with a short-acting neuromuscular blocking drug, or with a bolus of sodium thiopental, during such manipulations. Preventing the coughing and thrashing about that otherwise occurs in many of these patients helps to minimize the risk of inducing a huge ICP wave.

c. Cardiac Injury

Although it has been recognized for some time that blunt chest injury may be associated with damage to the heart, our experience shows that the association is very high — 50 to 60%. Usually, only a segment of the right heart wall is damaged, recovery is rapid, and critical reduction of cardiac output is unlikely. But when the cardiac septum and left ventricle are injured, a very significant reduction in cardiac hemodynamics may occur. We have had one adolescent die from traumatic heart failure, a girl whose brain injury was relatively minor.

d. Fulminant Neurogenic Pulmonary Edema (NPE)

This dreaded, fortunately uncommon, consequence of certain brain injuries that involve the hypothalamus can be a terrifying spectacle. Suddenly, the patient begins to produce a frothing, bloody pulmonary exudate that literally fills the tracheobronchial passages. Often they die within minutes. A volume-cycled ventilator is of help, along with a high oxygenation fraction, positive end-expiratory pressure (PEEP) and vigorous control of ICP. Occasionally, pharmaceutical blockade of the alpha-adrenergic SNS receptors seems to help.

More commonly, patients develop NPE of a less fulminant nature and over a longer interval. Early recognition of what's occurring, with institution of the above measures, can avert tragedy.

The caveat here is that PEEP of too high a value in such patients may aggravate an ICP problem by reducing venous outflow from the head. Obviously, the care of patients with NPE requires fine-tuning of therapy and unexcelled communication between physicians, nursing staff, and respiratory technologists.

In this chapter, we have examined the clinical spectrum of head injury in the context of the event and its immediate sequelae. Next, we shall turn our attention to the long-term effects of brain injury and, finally, to the principles of rehabilitation from head trauma.

SOURCES AND READINGS

Alexander E Jr, Davis CH Jr: Intra-uterine fracture of the infant's skull. *J Neurosurg, 30:*446-454, 1969.

Amacher AL, Li KT: Indirect trauma as a cause of acute infantile subdural hematomas. *Can Med Assoc J, 108:*1530, 1973.

Brink JD, Imbus C, Woo-Sam H: Physical recovery after severe closed head trauma in children and adolescents. *J Pediat, 97:*721-727, 1980.

Bruce DA, Schut L, Bruno LA, Wood JH, Sutton LN: Outcome following severe head injuries in children. *J Neurosurg 48:*679-688, 1978.

Hendrick EB, Harwood-Nash DCF, Hudson AR: Head injuries in children: a survey of 4465 consecutive cases at the Hospital for Sick Children, Toronto, Canada. *Clin Neurosurg, 11:*46-65, 1964.

Teasdale G, Jennett B: Assessment of coma and impaired consciousness. A practical scale. *Lancet, 2:*81-84, 1974.

CHAPTER 6

The Residuals of Head Injury

1. SPECIFIC NEUROLOGICAL DEFICITS

Even relatively minor head injuries occasionally cause a localized and specific neurological abnormality. Reference to Figure 10 will be useful for the discussion to follow. Fortunately, most such deficits are transient, resolving over periods of days, weeks, or months.

a. Oculomotor Nerve Palsies

If an oculomotor nerve is stretched and knocked out of action by the force of impact, it is usually the sixth cranial nerve. The sixth cranial nerve (abducens) is responsible for abduction of the eyeball (out-turning). The patient will experience double vision on lateral gaze. Small children frequently will suppress the double image, probably at a cortical level, or the offending eye may become amblyopic (functionally blind with both eyes open), for reasons that are not well understood. The older the patient, the more likely is the double vision to remain troublesome. One commonly observes that an afflicted person keeps one eye closed, usually the affected one, in order to avoid double vision. This symptom may be extremely upsetting to the patient, even to the point of nausea, vomiting, vertigo, and headache. Alternating a patch over one eye will prevent the double vision and the subjective symptoms, and will maintain visual acuity in both eyes.

Less commonly, the third cranial nerve (oculomotor nerve) is damaged at head impact. Then, the patient may experience double vision in all fields of gaze and even when the eyes are in the neutral position. Usually there is paralysis of the pupil, as well. When the pupil is fully dilated and non-reactive in the presence of normal ocular movement following trauma, a traumatic mydriasis is the common cause (see Chapter 5 section 3.a).

The fourth, or trochlear, nerve seldom is injured by impact. When it is, the complaint is of double vision when trying to focus downwards, particularly when going down stairs.

The oculomotor nerves, like all cranial nerves, are tethered at both ends. Sudden bouncing of the brain stem at head impact may put a stretch on the nerve that exceeds any natural slackness that is present. The abducens nerve has a very long passage from the pontine-medullary junction to the inferior lateral aspect of the cavernous sinus, within the subarachnoid space. It may be this long course that makes it so vulnerable to stretch.

b. Other Cranial Nerves

The only cranial nerves of which I personally have never seen a post-traumatic traction or compression injury are the ninth (glossopharyngeal) and the twelfth (hypoglossal), and even these occur, especially with crushing injuries of the skull. We have alluded to some aspects of specific cranial nerve injuries in Chapter 5 section 2.b.4, but further detail is apropos.

The olfactory (first) nerve may be avulsed during non-concussive injuries. Very recently, I was obliged to operate upon a ten-year-old girl who fell while skiing, fracturing her nose. She was not unconscious for even a moment. The nasal fracture was inconsequential, but she began to leak CSF from her nose, usually from the right nostril. This continued for six weeks, intermittently. Tomographic films of the anterior base of the skull failed to show any fractures. At operation, her right olfactory bulb had been torn away from the fine nerve filaments that pierce through the cribriform plate to the nasal cavity. Those filaments had withered, allowing CSF to leak through into the nose.

Damage to the optic (second) nerve usually occurs only in the context of major trauma to the orbit and its contents. Rarely, however, a less severe injury to the middle face and anterior skull base may produce a depressed fracture of the optic canal, compressing the optic nerve. Removal of the depressed fragment seldom is effective in restoring sight from that eye.

Injuries to the other cranial nerves (fifth, seventh, eighth, ninth, tenth, eleventh and twelfth) seldom occur as isolated entities. A basal fracture involving the petrous bone may disrupt the tiny bony ossicles of the middle ear, producing a conductive hearing loss. Or, the fracture may damage the inner ear hearing and balancing mechanisms; the acoustic and vestibular, and the seventh, nerves may be damaged alone or in any combination, especially if the fracture crosses the petrous bone very medially. Some patients may be vertiginous for several days following loss of the eighth nerve. Bilateral eighth nerve damage is a very serious disability indeed. Besides the total deafness, the patient is very unsure of equilibrium in the dark, particularly when traversing uneven terrain. It is most dangerous for this victim to try to swim underwater, because of complete loss of positional orientation in a near-zero gravity environment.

Crushing injuries of the skull may leave the patient with a devastating disability because of traction and avulsion injuries to many cranial nerves. Such deficits usually are permanent. Fortunately, these injuries are not common in children. They occur when the child's head is compressed relatively slowly, as when caught between a truck platform and a wall, or when run over on soft ground by a tire. During such low-velocity high-weight injuries, the entire petrous ridge may rotate, disrupting basal suture lines and tearing off cranial nerves one by one. The patient may not lose consciousness, may hear the skull cracking, and may recall the sequential loss of cranial nerve function as the injury progresses.

Facial injuries that crush the cheekbone frequently damage the second sensory division of the fifth nerve as it emerges just below the orbit. Sensory loss over the prominence of the cheek may be permanent. Upon occasion, a fracture of the horizontal ramus of the jaw may render the lower teeth and gum insensitive, often leading to premature loss of teeth.

c. Localized Motor Deficits

Bruising of cortical motor areas frequently produces a motor palsy, usually transient. But when the damage is more severe — for example, following laceration of the cortex by an indriven bone fragment — a permanent residual motor deficit may be the result. Cerebral cortical damage reduces the ability to initiate distal fine motor movement, often with an accompanying increase in motor tone, or spasticity. Extensive damage to the cortical motor areas of one hemisphere will be manifest as a contralateral hemiparesis or hemiplegia. The affected extremity is useful for ambulation and gross motor activities, but the fine, dexterous movements of the hand are lost. Occasionally, the patient continues to complain of a peculiar and subjective ease of fatiguability of an extremity for months and even years following cortical bruising. The explanation for this rather nebulous complaint is uncertain; it *may* be an indication of a significant reduction in the neuronal pool devoted to certain specific movements. Paralysis induced by seizure activity following trauma does *not* persist.

Damage in the deep cerebral motor nuclei — the basal ganglia — produces specific abnormalities of control of motor activity. The usual finding is a mixture of choreiform and athetoid movement, often made worse by excitement, tension, or prolonged activity. A writhing, sinuous movement of the arm may be seen, with short, jerky tics superimposed. If the muscles of the pharynx and larynx are involved, speech may become thick and garbled. Fortunately, these basal ganglia manifestations are rare as a residual of trauma. Principally, they are disorders of motor tone.

Injury to the subthalamic area of the brain stem may produce an extremely disabling movement disorder. I have seen it in five children, as their only readily discernible trauma residual. At rest, the extremity — usually the arm — is quiet and normal in appearance. With activity, however, the arm begins to jerk uncontrollably, even wildly. The arm may strike the patient in the face. Usually the excursions of the arm can be restrained by touching it or holding it lightly. This motor disorder is called *hemiballismus.*

Extensive damage to the cerebellum, especially if its deep nuclei are affected, may produce a permanent deficit in the proper coordination of motor activity, most obviously seen as poor control of the range and velocity of movement, acceleration and braking of an extremity in pursuit of a target, and difficulty in the organization of sequential movement. Cerebellar deficits often improve with time. A good example of a motor activity that may reveal subtle degrees of cerebellar injury is piano playing.

When cerebral cortical motor and deep nuclear motor damage has been diffuse and severe, an enormous spectrum of residual and permanent deficits may be seen, ranging from an overall mild reduction in fine motor skills through post-traumatic dystonic cerebral palsy to spastic tetraplegia. Since the pattern of motor damage varies with the individual, so do the manifestations.

d. Localized Sensory Deficits

These are rare following head injury in the absence of peripheral or cranial nerve, or spinal cord, trauma. Contusion in the thalamus may lead to a change in sensory appreciation in some area of the body, usually with a diffuse and unpleasant character. A crawling sensation, or a lingering hyperpathia may be experienced with the lightest of contact, over one half of the body or a more restricted area. Unfortunately, these symptoms may persist, and very often there is little to find on examination. The younger the patient, the less likely are such complaints.

e. Visual Deficits

Occasionally a concussive injury, even with only momentary loss of consciousness, will produce a transient blindness. It is probably brought on by direct impact forces, though vascular effects cannot be ruled out. Particularly for a child, the situation is terrifying. Parents are distraught at the prospect of permanent blindness, but the truth is that the symptoms are transient. Children with hydrocephalus and persisting large ventricular occipital horns are especially prone to this occurrence. In the latter, it is likely that a water-hammer effect is operational. Reassurance is all that is necessary, at least for the parents. The child may require mild sedation to control its terrified crying. Older children may appear to be acutely psychotic during the episode. In my experience, the blindness recedes in hours, very rarely one or two days.

We have discussed direct damage to an optic nerve previously. Field defects may result from secondary pressure effects such as occlusion of a posterior cerebral artery during expansion of an extracerebral clot, or from direct tissue-disruption as seen with deep cerebral contusions or hematomas. In the latter instance, the *optic radiations* — the fibre tracts passing from the lateral geniculate bodies to the visual primary cortex — are disrupted. In either case, some degree of contralateral field defect is permanent. It is extremely important to discover field defects; patients with such deficits cannot operate any sort of vehicle safely.

f. Specific Deficits in Higher Cortical Function

Extension damage to cortical language areas will result in permanent impairment of language mechanisms with one exception: an infant of less than three years or so should be able to tranfer language representation to the undamaged cerebral hemisphere. The clinical spectrum will vary, depending upon the surface topography of the injury. For example, permanent damage to both occipital lobes will interfere with all visually-based language functions. For such patients, it is important to document as accurately as possible the nature of the damage, as we shall see shortly.

Speech production, as distinct from language, may be affected adversely by deep motor nuclei and cerebellar injury. Respectively, the patient may exhibit garbled, thick, explosive speech, or a slow and scanning speech pattern.

Damage to the so-called non-dominant parietal lobe may cause permanent deficits in spacial conceptualization, orientation in one's envircnment, even in the emotional content and rhythm of language. Musical appreciation and performance may suffer following injury to the temporal lobe that is non-dominant for language. As evidence accumulates that the left hemisphere — at least in non-orientals — is *usually* dominant for analytical and language functions, while the right hemisphere dominates with respect to conceptualization, personal orientation, and emotional content of life — the "artistic" hemisphere — the role of professionals expert in the study of delineation of deficits, post-traumatic or otherwise, grows ever more important and interesting. For children in their formative educational and psychological years, access to neuropsychologists and to therapists of all sorts may be crucial to their prognosis.

Injury to the corpus callosum, connecting as it does analagous anatomical cortical areas of the two hemispheres, may result in important *disconnection syndromes.* A good clinical example here is the disconnection of the cortical visual association areas that may occur with severe damage to the posterior corpus callosum, the splenium. Visual language information entering the right hemisphere from the left visual field must be transferred to the left hemisphere visual association areas before it can be interpreted as language. The patient with severe damage in the splenium must learn to swing his eyes far to the left — thus putting the words on a page into his right visual field, hence, left hemisphere, or he will be unable to read the left side of a page.

Intellect is a measure of the integrated activity of the entire cerebral cortex and the integrity of the cortical connections. In general, the extent of intellectual damage following trauma is proportional to the volume of brain destroyed. Many of the features of intellect and personality have to do with more widely distributed brain functions such as learning and behavior, to be discussed next.

2. BEHAVIORAL PROBLEMS

Following diffuse brain injury, parents will remark often that the child is "different" somehow. A previously aggressive child may seem much more placid; a boy formerly quiet and studious may become extroverted and supercilious. Sometimes, particularly in adolescents, there emerges a sociopathic streak, even a psychopathic tendency. It is as though a social inhibitory force has been dispelled. One mother told me that her teenage son acted as though he had lost his conscience.

Post-traumatic behavioral abnormalities are common following diffuse injury to the frontal lobes, especially the under surfaces. The frontal lobes have much to do with such psychological traits as judgment, impulse control, social behavior, appropriate reactions, motivation — all those features that make social interactions among humans tolerable. The patient with a severe post-traumatic behavioral disorder is all the more poignant and tragic because usually he is unaware of the extent of his problem. His family certainly is not unaware, and their grief may be profound as they contemplate the future for a child who may require social and behavioral supervision for years. How tragic to watch an adolescent girl, retaining her motor skills, her learning ability, her good looks, become an utterly promiscuous social outcast because of lack of judgment and impulse control. Such residuals of head injury are catastrophic to the individual, particularly when accompanied by even minor reductions in intellectual capacity. Seldom are such behavioral abnormalities discerned before the patient leaves the hospital; they become apparent as the child or teenager resumes previous environmental and social contacts. Sometimes the situation improves over weeks or months, sometimes it does not. Parents usually notice a change in sibling relationships, then hear of troubles that the child is having in school or in other social contacts. A "mean streak" may emerge, particularly towards younger and smaller children. Indifference to social graces is common, and language inhibitions may evaporate entirely. Parents and others may be embarrassed but tolerant to begin with, then frustrated, angry, and annoyed, then recriminatory. I have known children to be thrown out of school as punishment for this socially unacceptable, inappropriate behavior, of course to no effect. Such children need patient, understanding therapy, not reprisal.

Very occasionally, following a mild concussion, a child may become acutely psychotic for hours or days. One of my patients, a girl, did so twice at ages nine and thirteen. On each occasion she was unconscious for only seconds. She showed a thoroughly disordered thought pattern and vivid hallucinations, resolving over three or four days. Whether or not such reactions to head trauma carry any foreboding of psychiatric disorder in later life is unknown.

3. LEARNING DISABILITIES

We come now to a subject of extraordinary importance. Only within the past few — very few — years has the reality and extent of post-traumatic learning disability become recognized among the neurologists, neurosurgeons, neuropsychologists and therapists who care for head-injured children. In general, the more diffuse the damage, the more severe and lingering the effects upon learning capacity. But even so-called trivial head injuries may have a significant effect upon memory mechanisms.

We must digress briefly at this point, into the intricate circuitry and anatomy associated with memory, at least as it is understood at the moment. Learning, of course, cannot occur in the absence of memory. The study of learning disorders, then, devolves upon an understanding of memory mechanisms.

Anatomically, the brain structures that are known to play some role in the permanent imprinting or in the recall of memory are: the medial temporal lobes, especially the hippocampi and related areas; the dorsal-medial thalamic nuclei; the mamillary bodies below the hypothalamus; certain fibre tracts connecting these structures to one another and to other cortical areas, such as the fornices (hippocampus to mammillary bodies, hence to thalamus), and other fine tracts coursing through the deep midline diencephalon and midbrain. Permanent damage to both medial temporal lobes has a devastating effect upon memory mechanisms, hence upon learning.

Current concepts about how memories are formed are still being enlarged and refined. When new information enters the system, it circulates as sensory neuronal impulses for at least a few seconds, probably not minutes, and it is very vulnerable to extinction. This "sensory" phase sometimes is referred to as immediate memory. Because no anatomical imprinting has occurred yet, extinction or cancellation of such information easily is effected by concussion, anesthetic agents, even by competition from other information being received and processed simultaneously. This may explain why so many patients are amnestic for the events immediately (several seconds) preceding a mild concussion.

Beyond this point the theories are more properly classified as hypotheses. Two aspects of memory must be accounted for, the imprinting of memory and the recall of memory.

For years, so-called recent memory was thought to consist of myriad electrical circuits operating continuously. In that case, any event — such as severe hypothermia or large doses of thiopental — that can produce electrical silence in the brain should wipe out all recent, non-anatomical, memory. Of course, this does not occur. Then, the famous flat worm experiment came along. If one trains those little beasts to travel safely through a maze by avoidance conditioning, then grinds up the little dears and injects the extract into unconditioned flatworms, the new batch learns the maze much more quickly than did their cannibalized cousins. This indicated that *something*, be it physical or chemical, is capable of transferring memory.

Suffice it to say here that the current paradigm is that memory imprinting involves a change in the structure and number of synaptic contacts within appropriate neuronal pools, perhaps in the structure of cell membranes and of some intracellular organelles such as ribosomes. This is a fascinating field of research at the basic and clinical levels, and an impressive literature is developing very rapidly.

The imprinting of memory takes time, it seems. Recall of or reencounter with the same sensory information within an appropriately short interval reinforces and accelerates the process. The longer the interval between reinforcements, the less likely is the memory to become permanent or to be easily recalled. Obviously, a memory cannot be recalled if it was not imprinted in the first place.

As every student soon realizes, learning can be improved by good concentration upon new information, and by repetition. Of recent years, neuropsychologists have pointed out that individuals vary with respect to the information modality that is used most efficiently in learning. Some people do better from auditory information, some from visual. Children — anyone, for that matter — who have sustained permanent damage to, say, visual association and language areas will run into unsurmountable obstacles when trying to learn from language information presented visually. In the ideal, such a child's problem would be identified quickly by a good neuropsychologist, and a learning program stressing auditory perception and skills would be instituted. Unfortunately, ideals seldom are realized.

Some information seems to become well imprinted, but if not recalled at intervals, fades and then disappears from memory. Other information becomes inprinted so firmly that it can be recalled even after years of neglect — such as regimental numbers or names of certain long-departed childhood friends. Memory of the patterns of fine motor activities seems to persist as well, even if not used for long periods, though the expert coordination necessary to do the procedure well may take time to recapture. An example here is reacquisition of skill at the piano. In this context, relearning of forgotten material to a firmly-imprinted, familiar level usually takes less time and effort the second time around — as though the memory remained in fact, but the mechanisms for its recall deteriorated. Permanent — formerly referred to as long-term memory — appears to involve the entire cerebral cortex, at least as far as storage is concerned.

How memories are recalled is uncertain. Familiar information springs to mind immediately upon demand, while less-used memories require an interval of searching. All of us have had the experience of trying to remember a name or a fact, being unable to do so, only to have the information occur to mind suddenly sometime later even though the circumstances may be inappropriate. It is as though the search circuitry must be recruited, perhaps reinforced, even reestablished, before the desired information can be recalled.

In any event, learning will be compromised by interference with either the process of imprinting or of recall, or any admixture of the two. That head injury severe enough to alter consciousness for days or weeks regularly affects learning ability is a long-recognized fact. The great revelation regarding the clinical residua of head injury over the past few years has been that even mild — so-called trivial — concussion may do the same thing. A child sustaining head impact with loss of consciousness of only seconds, or none at all, may experience significant difficulty in new information processing and recall for several days, weeks, even months. And if he or she has another concussion within or even after that interval of learning impairment, the effects are more than additive. Brief concussive episodes can and do cause permanent anatomical damage to the brain areas concerned with learning. Successive concussions have a cumulative effect upon the brain. These facts are incontrovertible. We have alluded to this problem in Chapter 3, and in the case of severely head-injured patients in Chapter 5 section 3.e. Now it is time for serious, perhaps unwelcome, comment relating to school-aged children and organized sport.

Any sport in which the head is a target or is used as an offensive weapon embodies, as an inherent risk of the sport, a high incidence of concussion. My approach to the problem is: if the patient has been unconscious, or has been confused and disoriented for several minutes or hours, he should not play that or any related sport for at least six weeks — some would say, one year. After two concussions, he or she should give up the sport. This approach, of course, is centered upon the welfare of the athlete and intellectual capacity, not upon the good of the team or the patient's potential ability in the sport. Coaches and organizers of high school or other teams and sports find this attitude outrageous, very often. Of course, the older athlete is free to choose, but he must be appraised of the risks. But for children, quite simply, the stakes are too high. One has only to see a couple of high school football stars who have suffered four or five concussions and whose knees have been damaged by violent maneuvers to begin to realize that something tantamount to child abuse has been occurring. Harsh words, perhaps, but true.

In my experience, the curricula that are most likely to suffer following head injury are math-related subjects, secondary languages, and motor activities requiring highly coordinated, rapid finger movement such as typing. A drop in grades of one or two levels is not uncommon at least for that semester. Learning disabilities following head injury are very real, and very important.

4. THE POST-TRAUMATIC SYNDROME

This peculiar affliction that may linger for weeks or months after a minor head injury has baffled clinicians for years. Fortunately, it occurs rarely in young children, but its frequency increases during adolescence. Some consider the symptoms to reflect a functional or neurotic disorder; I do not, because the complaints are so stereotyped and the course so typical. I have no idea why it settles like a fog upon some individuals and not upon others, nor why the incidence seems higher among patients with milder injuries.

The post-traumatic syndrome (PTS) usually begins several days after the head injury. The patient complains of headache, usually dull, constant and of medium to low intensity. Accompanying the headache is photophobia, sensitivity to sound, irritability and short temper — particularly with siblings — inability to concentrate, day-dreaming, and an ill-defined lassitude and ennui that resembles depression. Neurological examination and fundi are normal. If done, EEG and CT scan are normal. The patient and parents are alarmed; reassurance of recovery is essential. I have learned to tell the patient and families that the symptoms are real, although their etiology is not understood; that there is nothing of ominous import occurring intracranially; that the symptoms will vanish in time; that they should resume normal activities, and that they should use the least and simplest of analgesics. The results have been gratifying.

It is axiomatic that when symptoms of PTS are associated with (1) any evidence of raised intracranial pressure — such as papilledema, or headache that wakes from sleep or is accompanied by vomiting or acute exacerbation with coughing, straining or bending over, — (2) any neurological deficits, and (3) seizures, prompt investigation is required. The CT scan usually is most efficient in this regard.

5. EPILEPSY

We have discussed some aspects of this topic in Chapter 5 section 2.c, especially in regards to seizures occurring within seconds to days following head injury.

Epilepsy means a recurrent and refractory seizure disorder. The likelihood of post-traumatic epilepsy (PTE) occurring is related to the type and extent of initial injury. Dirty, penetrating wounds of the skull and brain carry a risk of PTE of nearly 50%, whereas simple concussive injuries will lead to PTE in less than 1% of cases. Between these extremes, the presence of permanent cortical or white matter injury — particularly in or near motor cortex — an inherent seizure tendency, a late-onset mass lesion, or anterior and medial temporal lobe injury, increase the risk of PTE. By whatever means, a focus of unusually irritable neurones develops, capable of triggering a seizure and of recruiting other neurones into the seizure discharge. These foci often are associated with a glial, reparative scar in the cortex. The injury itself, or the scarring later, may cause significant interruption of the incoming fibres to a group of neurones. If most of the interrupted incoming signals were inhibitory in nature, our proposed neuronal pool may become hyperexcitable. Other factors that may be involved include unusual local chemical fluxes caused by the abnormal number of glial cells, and anomalies in local regulation of blood flow. Whatever the cause, a seizure discharge begins, spreads, and becomes manifest clinically.

PTE often has a focal onset clinically with rapid secondary generalization, and it may be very difficult to control. Meticulous debridement of penetrating wounds of the brain, particularly the removal of foreign material, proved of value in reducing the incidence of PTE in battle casualties. The prophylactic use of anticonvulsants has not been proven to be effective in aborting the onset of PTE, though common clinical practice is to place likely candidates on such drugs for three to six months post-traumatically, then slowly weaning them if no seizures have occurred.

When a seizure focus can be identified by sophisticated EEG techniques, it may be excisable surgically. Such procedures usually are carried out under local anesthesia, using direct recording from the cortex to identify the boundaries of the focus.

Occasionally, the post-traumatic seizure disorder may originate from deep in the temporal lobes, even the upper brainstem. Then, its manifestations may be those of (1) *temporal lobe epilepsy*, with complex automatisms, hallucinatory aura, behavioral abnormalities, even absence attacks, or (2) *partial motor seizures*, where paroxysmal episodes of blankness, staring unawareness, or collapse may predominate. Sometimes, the possibility that a patient may be suffering from these forms of PTE must be considered when he or she presents as a behavior or learning disorder that has a fluctuating pattern to it.

6. LATE RECOGNITION OF ANATOMICAL PATHOLOGY

Sometimes I am asked to see a youngster several months, even years after a head injury because of the onset of a headache problem, a new or increased neurological deficit, a slippage in school performance, a seizure, or some combination thereof. The neurological work-up of such a case may reveal surprising pathology, the anatomy of which most often is:

a. Hydrocephalus

Even with minor head bumps, blood may be spilled into the subarachnoid space. Sometimes, the subarachnoid blood elicits sufficient inflammatory reaction and subsequent scarring to interfere with proper circulation of the CSF. Even a minor imbalance in the amount of CSF produced compared to the amount absorbed each day will, in time, cause ventricular enlargement, or hydrocephalus. Correction of the intracranial CSF dynamics by placement of a CSF shunt usually is beneficial.

There is significant caveat here. Severe, diffuse brain injury may result in a significant degree of brain atrophy, with ventricular enlargement on the basis of volume loss from the hemispheres. In such cases, a CT scan will show "hydrocephalus," and in addition, shrinkage of the cortical gyri with greatly enlarged sulci filled with CSF, on the brain surface. Placing a shunt in such a situation will not help at all.

The symptoms and signs of slowly progressive hydrocephalus frequently are slight and subtle at first. Headache, evidence of raised ICP such as papilledema or split skull sutures, and deterioration in school (or other) performance are the usual harbingers. Seizures may occur.

b. Calcified Subdural Hematoma

Sometimes the membranes that surround a chronic subdural hematoma become calcified, even ossified. At that stage, the hematoma is not acting as a space-occupying mass. The child may or may not have a fixed neurological deficit from the time of the original injury. Figure 37 is an example.

Often these lesions are discovered incidentally on skull radiographs, but they may induce seizures. There is a very significant risk of causing further damage to the cerebral cortex if one attempts to remove the calcified membrane. Seizure control usually can be effected with anticonvulsant medications.

Years ago, chronic bilateral subdurals were a fairly common finding in young infants admitted to hospital because of failure to thrive, seizures, or simply for investigation of a big head. Some of these may have been due to birth injury or child abuse, but in most cases the etiology was unknown. It is uncertain why they are seen less commonly now; perhaps better nutrition, better

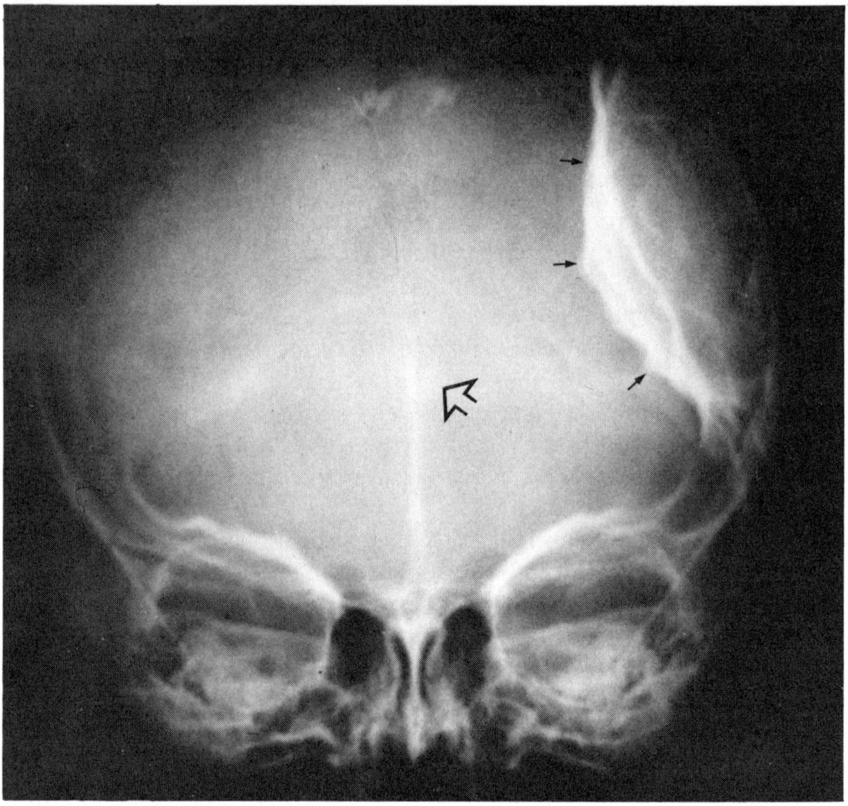

Figure 37. Towne's projection of skull, showing calcified chronic subdural (arrows at edge of calcified membrane). The open arrow indicates a calcified pineal gland. Note that it is shifted slightly to the side of the calcified mass. This patient had a right hemiparesis, and atrophy of the left cerebral hemisphere.

therapy for gastroenteritis and dehydration, better perinatal care, all contribute.

c. Porencephaly

This term literally means "a hole in the brain." In the context of trauma, a porencephalic cyst usually represents the residual cavity of an intracerebral hematoma. The cyst may communicate with the ventricle, or with the surface subarachnoid space.

The tendency is for such a cyst to enlarge with time, slowly compressing surrounding white matter and causing an ingavescent neurological deficit, seizures, or headaches. Drainage of the cyst by means of a shunt is beneficial.

d. Retained Bone Chips or Foreign Objects

If these objects are left behind after debridement and repair of a penetrating or perforating injury to the brain, they may become the nidus for scar or cyst formation, or for abscess formation if the bone or metal fragment is contaminated with microorganisms. The process may take months or years to reach the point of causing symptoms of raised ICP, neurological deficit, or seizures. Excision of such lesions may be difficult technically, and risky. Obviously, prevention is the best therapy.

In this chapter, we have covered some of the aspects of the residuals of head injury. Clearly, even mild concussion may have lingering and significant consequences. The more severe the injury to the brain, the more likely are there to be permanent disabilities. Overall, the loss of human potential following brain trauma is a tragedy of major proportions.

SOURCES AND READINGS

Barondes SH, Squire LR: Time and the biology of memory. *Clin Neurosurg, 19:*381-396, 1972.

Fuld PA, Fisher P: Recovery of intellectual ability after closed head injury. *Develop Med Child Neurol, 19:*495-502, 1977.

Geshwind N: Disconnexion syndromes in animals and man. Part 1. *Brain, 88:* 237-294, 1965.

Gronwall D, Wrightson P: Delayed recovery of intellectual function after minor head injury. *Lancet, 2:*605-609, 1974.

Gronwall D, Wrightson P: Cumulative effect of concussion. *Lancet, 2:*995-997, 1975.

Hugenholtz H, Richard MT: Return to athletic competition following concussion, *Can Med Assoc J, 127:*827-829, 1982.

Jennett, B: Post-traumatic epilepsy. In: *Handbook of Clinical Neurology,* Vol. 24. North Holland Publishing Co., Amsterdam, 1976.

Klonoff H, Low MD, Clark C: Head injuries in children: a prospective five year follow-up. *J Neurol Neurosurg Psychiat, 40:*1211-1219, 1977.

Levin HS, Eisenberg HM: Neuropsychological outcome of closed head injury in children and adolescents. *Child's Brain, 5:*281-292, 1979.

Milner B: Disorders of learning and memory after temporal lobe lesions in man. *Clin Neurosurg, 19:*421-446, 1972.
Podoshin L, Fradis M: Hearing loss after head injury. *Arch Otolaryngol, 101:* 15-18, 1975.
Pribham KH: Neurological investigations of the associative structure of memory. *Clin Neurosurg, 19:*397-420, 1972.
Schneider RC, McGillicuddy JE: Concomitant craniocerebral and spinal trauma with special reference to the cervicomedullary junction. In: *Handbook of Clinical Neurology.* Vol. 24, pp. 141-177. P.J. Vinken and G.W. Bruyn, Eds. North Holland Publishing Co., Amsterdam, 1976.
Shulman K: Late complications of head injuries in children. *Clin Neurosurg, 19:*371-380, 1972.
Yarnell PR, Lynch S: The "ding": amnestic states in football trauma. *Neurology (Minneap), 23:*196-197, 1973.
Young B, Rapp RP, Norton JA, Haack D, Tibbs PA, Bean JR: Failure of prophylactically administered phenytoin to prevent early post-traumatic seizures. *J Neurosurg, 58:*231-235, 1983.
Ibid., pp. 236-241.

CHAPTER 7

Prevention and Rehabilitation

1. PREVENTION

It is ridiculous to imagine that all head injuries might be prevented. To do so would require the incarceration of all children and adolescents in impenetrable foam–filled cavities, underground. Children *will* continue to climb onto and fall off of things, get into scraps, play risky games, ride vehicles of various kinds, and so on. Nevertheless, there are some things that can be done, most of them pure common sense.

In the home, staircases can be guarded and items that lure toddlers into climbing can be set elsewhere. Certain playthings such as lawn darts — they penetrate a thin skull very nicely indeed — can be forbidden.

Car seats are essential for infants, but to be effective, they must be fixed to rigid structures. Many jurisdictions now legislate the use and type of such devices. There are well–designed head gear available for cyclists, and their proper use will reduce significantly the severity of head injury from cycling accidents.

Personally, I cannot imagine why parents would allow a child to participate in the "sport" of boxing. Headgear will *not* protect the brain when the blow lands on the face, as most do. Only the outlawing of blows to the head will make that sport safe. The same comments apply to full–contact martial arts.

American–style football accounts for more athletic injuries, including head injuries, than all other team sports combined. The search for effective headgear has been the lonely quest of Professor Schneider at Ann Arbor, but it is the tactics of the game that maim and kill. Using the top of the helmet as a ram, as in spearing a ball–carrier, is extraordinarily dangerous. Vertical motion of the brain and brain stem within the skull may produce a point of impaction at the junction of the medulla and the upper cervical spinal cord, because the cord is tethered laterally to the dura by the dentate ligaments, and is not as free to move vertically as is the medulla. A tiny hemorrhage may occur at this level, deep within the cord, producing sudden respiratory paralysis: a high price to pay for stopping a running back.

It is a truism that protective equipment may have the opposite effect of what was intended. Boxing gloves allow blows to be struck with much greater force; the padding in the gloves does nothing to protect the brain. Football helmets and pads provide a very false sense of security. The wearer supposes that he may now fling himself about with utter abandon, and the gear will protect him. Rugger is a rough game resembling football, played without protective equipment of any sort, yet the incidence of serious head, neck and joint injuries is much less than in the American game. Only when parents, educators and coaches become aware of the consequences of head injury will the prevalence of sports-related concussion decline.

There is simply no excuse for not wearing seat belts while riding within a vehicle. Most serious head injuries in survivable motor vehicle accidents occur because of secondary impacts within or without the vehicle. Arguments against compulsory seat belt usage based upon personal liberty are valid politically and philosophically, but they do not protect the brain, either. Perhaps more compliance with seat belt usage could be accomplished by the insurance companies, if they refused to compensate victims who were not wearing their belts.

Obviously, if the head injury does not occur, there are no residuals. We shall never reduce the incidence of head injury to zero, because risk is a part of the human condition. We can, however, make some inroad into the epidemic proportions of the problem as it exists now.

2. REHABILITATION

After the fact, we are left with the challenge of making optimum the remaining abilities of the patient, and of finding new ways for the victim to do and learn things.

During the past decade, facilities and techniques for the after-care and retraining of head- and spinal cord-injured patients have improved by orders of magnitude. Now, many institutions have very sophisticated programs in place. Victims and their families form associations for advancing the cause of the disabled. Increasingly, emphasis is placed upon the abilities of the victims, not their disabilities. Within the community, awareness of the needs of neurologically disabled people has increased; curb ramps, properly equipped washrooms, special transports — all are manifestations. Many children's rehabilitation centers now combine the rehab program with education, to the convenience of all. Gradually, the old fiction that disabled children are, by definition, retarded children is being dispelled.

Programs for the rehabilitation of neurologically-injured patients may be run very conveniently in association with programs for neurological disability caused by congenital malformations, cerebral palsy, and the like. It is always better to concentrate the talents of the allied health professionals as much as possible.

Rehabilitation of the neurologically-injured child should begin on the ward, even while the state of consciousness remains altered. Baseline physical evaluations can be done, along with therapy to prevent joint malpositions and muscle contractures. There is never an excuse for the development of decubitus ulcers these days. They are signs of improper nursing techniques and inadequate nutritional support.

Further on nutrition: within a week of injury, should the child be unable to resume full oral intake, a nutritional expert should be enlisted to supervise the problem. This issue is critical for children who remain in an altered state of consciousness for two weeks or more. Caloric and protein support is essential, preferably given by the gastrointestinal tract. Loss of more than 30% of lean body mass probably is irreplaceable. Severely head- or cord-injured patients frequently have an exaggerated early post-traumatic catabolic response, and fat stores may appear to literally melt away during the first two or three weeks. Expert advice on the preparation and administration of food-stuffs that will prevent excessive loss of lean body mass is available easily to any unit that looks after these patients.

A comprehensive program for the rehabilitation of neurologically disabled children incorporates all of the people and services listed in Table 5. It works very well if such a program, with its clinics, its outreach programs, its community focus, can be connected physically with a Children's Rehabilitation Center, or whatever it might be called. There must be a medical director for the program, most appropriately a developmental pediatrician or a

TABLE 5
A POST-HEAD INJURY REHABILITATION PROGRAM

Medical	*Allied Health Professional*
Orthopedics	Physiotherapy
Developmental Pediatrics	Occupational Therapy
Neurology/Neurosurgery	Speech Therapy
Dental/Facial	Psychometrics
ENT	Neuropsychology
Ophthalmology	Nutrition
Physical Medicine	Nursing
Urodynamics	Education
Plastics	Seating/Bracing
	Social Work
	Transport

physiatrist. A very useful adjunct for the administration of such a program is an advisory committee chosen from the allied health professionals, upon whom the success of the program depends.

Rehabilitation from severe brain injury is a long, slow process. The patient may make striking progress for a few weeks, then level off or even slip back a little, then surge forward again, and so on. The whole thing often is frustrating for parents and therapists, and at times it may be difficult to avoid conveying a sense of discouragement to the child. Noticeable progress is likely to continue for at least three years in children, perhaps longer. Also, the patient's inherent motor skills — from undamaged areas — are increasing with age. Much of the therapy for these little victims is aimed at circumventing specific disabilities. Of course, residual deficits in intellectual function compromise the final outcome in direct proportion to the deficit.

At one end of the spectrum we have the child with a perceptual handicap that may or may not resolve. He requires an individual educational program and patience. At the other extreme is the totally dependent, even vegetative survivor of an incredible tragedy, the loss of his or her promise of achievement and humanity. His presence reminds us that head injury is not at all funny. The destruction done to young lives and the everlasting tragedy visited upon their families is a national sorrow. It behooves us, each of us, to do what we can to help.

A national organization has been formed by families of the head-injured, the patients themselves, and professionals concerned with the plight of the victims of head trauma. The goals of the National Head Injury Foundation* (NHIF) are: (1) to increase awareness throughout our society of the extent of the problem, (2) to provide information regarding available resources for victims and families, (3) to develop a support network for victims and families, and (4) encourage and establish specialized head injury rehabilitation programs. Such an effort is long overdue, and as has happened previously with other crippling conditions, the impetus for organization has come from the families of victims. Chapters exist in most states and in many communities. In conjunction with the increasing number of good rehabilitation programs available in more communities, progress is being made. There is yet a long way to go.

SOURCES AND READINGS

Gurdjian ES: Prevention and mitigation of injuries. *Clin Neurosurg, 19:*43-57, 1972.

Schneider RC: *Head and Neck Injuries in Football: Mechanisms, Treatment, and Prevention.* Williams and Wilkins, Baltimore, 1973.

---

* Information concerning the NHIF is available from The National Head Injury Foundation, 280 Singletary Lane, Framingham, MA 01701.

Index

H

I

L

M

N

O

P

R

S

T

V

X

MARY ELLEN HAYDEN, PH.D.
PATE REHABILITATION ENDEAVORS, INC.